What people are saying

M000191940

"The book 'Eating To Die' is an easy-to-read resource for having a healthy life. In a culturally sensitive manner, it provides useful information and suggestions to African Americans on how to make significant lifestyle changes."

Clarice Pyles, R.N., B.S., M.S.

"This is a most effective book. It will appeal to persons who are most in need of Lottie's insights and delightfully written suggestions for healthy living."

Dr. Marie Branch, R.N., M.A., D.C.

"After reading 'Eating to Die' I learned that no matter what my health condition is, I could do better if I eat healthier, and stop smoking. I celebrated my first week without smoking after reading this book. Thank you, Lottie."

Nedra Anthony, Poet

"For many years, I watched my friend Lottie as she picked her way tediously through the darkness of self-destructive behavior, into the light of a very healthy lifestyle change – a metamorphosis. And now, with this book, she has lovingly dropped bread crumbs for us to follow, and gain a way into the light of healthy living".

Patricia Jackson, L.V.N.

To: Sheila Reid,

I wish for your the

very best of health.

Dr. Lottie Perkins

Eating To Die

Changing African American
Attitudes About Health

Eating
To Die

Changing African American
Attitudes About Health

Lottie Perkins, R.N., B.S.N., M.H.A.

MILLIGAN BOOKS   BOOKS   CALIFORNIA

Printed and Bound in the United States of America
Published and Distributed by:
Milligan Books, Inc.

Editing by Karyn L. Wilkening, *Expert Editing, Ink.*, San Diego, CA
Book coaching by Sheryl Mallory-Johnson
Cover Layout by Kevin Allen
Formatting by Caldonia Joyce

First Printing, September 2007
10987654321

ISBN: 978-0-9799308-6-7

Milligan Books
1425 W. Manchester Blvd., Suite C
Los Angeles, CA 90047

www.milliganbooks.com
drrosie@aol.com
(323) 750-3592

This book is dedicated to my children
Rosalind, Thelma, Edward, and Sheryl;
and to my beloved sister *Georgene,*
who inspired many lives.

Contents

Acknowledgments

I am grateful to many people who contributed to this book. My special thanks to those who took the time and effort to read my manuscript and provide me with invaluable feedback: Sheryl Mallory-Johnson, for her skillful book coaching; Clarice Pyles, R.N., B.A., M.S,. for her human perspective; Patricia Jackson L.V.N., for her practical perspective; Nedra Anthony, poet, for her personal perspective; and Dr. Marie Branch, R.N., M.A., D.C., for her historical perspective, and vast knowledge of health.

My gratitude to Dr. Lorraine Johnson, Ph.D., L.C.S.W., for her words of encouragement; Dr. Rosie Milligan, who has encouraged me to write for many years; and Karyn Wilkening, for the expert editing of my manuscript.

Heartfelt thanks to my beloved parents, George and Telia Williams, who stood by me with love through my turbulent years and taught me the value of independence and entrepreneurship; my wonderful children, Rosalind, Thelma, Edward, and Sheryl; my siblings, Clarice, Renee, and Daniel, for their continuous love and support, and my beloved siblings, Tony, Harold, and Georgene, who are always with me in spirit; my nephew, Ruben, for his sweet concern about my well-being; my friend Sandra, for her support; and Sister Ana, my beloved surrogate mother, who taught me the value of prayer.

Krishnamurti

"If you are here
merely to have confirmation,
to be encouraged in your thinking,
then your listening has little meaning.
But, if you are listening to find out,
then your mind is free,
not committed to anything;
it is very acute, sharp, alive, inquiring,
curious, and therefore capable of
discovery."

Introduction

African Americans are dying, and in many instances, dying younger than any other ethnic group. This reality profoundly disturbs me—and inspired me to write this book. After watching the health of my family, friends, co-workers, and patients deteriorate, I was emotionally drained. I wanted to understand why we as African Americans would not, or did not, take better care of ourselves. Too many of us are stricken with life threatening illnesses, or are debilitated because of poor diets, harmful customs, mismanagement of medical problems, and a complete lack of commitment to exercise.

In my search to determine why African Americans have such a callous attitude about their health, I discovered that the answer was not simply that we do not care about our health, but that there are historical, emotional, psychological, and social factors that hinder us from taking steps to improve our quality of life through proper health management. I will provide factual case studies that illustrate how our destructive health behaviors, rationalization, and denial can lead to illness, disability, and death.

However, despite our destructive health behaviors, I know that we have the power to change our circumstances. This is why I am on a mission to help African Americans become proactive about their health by providing healthy lifestyle strategies to eliminate our destructive behavior and attitudes.

These strategies are based partly on my own personal health program. I do not encourage people to do anything that I do not do myself. In other words, *I practice what I preach.*

For more than thirty years, through health consultations, lectures and classes that I instruct, I have talked about the importance of healthy eating, exercising regularly, and taking time to relax. The immense benefits I have received from my personal health program compel me to share it with others.

As African Americans, we have traversed the seas under the worst circumstances, survived the greatest hardships, and turned misfortune into prosperity, but we are not done.

Hopefully the culturally-specific information contained in these pages will not only help us to value our freedom, but also to value our health—mind, body, and spirit—and help us to learn how to EAT TO LIVE versus EATING TO DIE.

I am confident that the health and lifestyle of African Americans *can change for the better.*

This book is my contribution toward that effort.

Lottie Mallory-Perkins

*"No one
is here to stay,
so...
quality of life
is the only way."*

PART I

CHOOSING QUALITY OF LIFE

CHAPTER 1

Playing Russian Roulette with Your Health

Russian Roulette is a deadly game. You literally point a gun at your head and pull the trigger, not knowing if there is a bullet in the chamber that will blow your brains out. One chance in six you'll die; five chances in six you'll live. Either way, your odds of survival are slim.

Living a life of destructive eating and lifestyle habits is as dangerous as putting a gun to your head. What you are doing is increasing your odds of developing a serious illness that will lead to an early death.

3

There was a time when I played Russian Roulette with my life. As a matter of fact, I could have been a "poster child" for the game. At age sixteen I had my first child, and by the time I was twenty-one, I had four children and was in an abusive marriage. I smoked a pack of cigarettes a day, drank alcohol, and was one of many who smoked marijuana during the 1960's. I assumed that as long as I eliminated pork from my diet and ate a few vegetables a week, I wasn't at risk. I was deceiving myself.

Given my family history of chronic diseases, had I not put down the self-destructive revolver when I was in my thirties, *I probably wouldn't be alive today.*

The first change I made was to flee my abusive marriage, which meant raising four children alone. You may not be surprised that a major part of my early adult years were difficult, extremely stressful, and depressing.

Facing the harsh reality that I couldn't care sufficiently for four children on minimum wages, I went back to school to pursue a higher education. Taking care of four young children and going to school was a constant daily struggle, and by the ripe old age of thirty-one, I was burned out.

Something had to give, and I didn't want it to be my health. I knew that in order to handle the pace of my hectic life, as well as maintain a healthy mental and emotional state, *I had to change.*

The lifestyle changes I made weren't easy and didn't happen overnight. It was a process that gradually evolved into my present lifestyle of healthy eating, exercise, prayer, and meditation.

I'm often asked why I decided to make drastic changes. I find this question peculiar. It's like asking why

4

did I decide to be healthy, why did I decide to cherish the body/temple God gave me, why did I decide to live for my children, or why did I decide to live instead of die?

The reasons for changing my lifestyle were quite simple. I wanted to be healthy, look my best, and live to see my children and grandchildren grow up. I wanted to increase the quality of my life.

Choosing a healthier lifestyle was the best decision I could have made. I have more energy, my overall health has improved, and I look and feel much younger than my calendar years.

Do you think that you need to make a lifestyle change? If you're not sure, ask yourself these questions:

- Do I feel well most of the time?
- Do I have healthy eating habits? Or does my diet consist of fried chicken, burgers and fries, snack foods and sweets?
- Do I take care of my medical problems?
- Do I exercise enough?
- Do I take time out to relax?
- Do I have energy and vitality?
- Do I look and feel older than my calendar years?

If, after asking yourself these questions, you're still not sure, think about how many times you've clicked the self-destructive revolver and prayed that the bullet wouldn't kill you. Where do you get your ammunition on a daily basis? Is it from a poor diet, lack of exercise, alcohol, drugs, or not managing your medical problems?

Will your bullet eventually lead to heart disease, hypertension, diabetes, or kidney failure? Obesity? Or cancer?

I want to help you put down that revolver. It might involve scaring you a bit with ugly facts and case examples... but please remember my intention is to make you aware of the personal power and the options you have to improve your health and your life.

Turn the page.

Don't be afraid.

You can do it!

Lottie Mallory-Perkins

*"We may not have control
over our QUANTITY of life,
but we do have control
over our QUALITY of life."*

CHAPTER 2

The Choice of Quality

As if it were yesterday, I can vividly recall the day that severe complications from Type II diabetes hospitalized my sister. The deep emotional pain I experienced was torturous. I stood next to her bed and stroked her beautiful hair, which, amazingly, had less salt than pepper for a woman of sixty-three.

Only five years earlier my sister had been healthy and vibrant. She was an entrepreneur directing a successful nurse assistant training program, an evangelist whose ministry had grown tremendously, and a real estate broker—all before this disease left her speechless, totally blind, in kidney failure, and suffering from a massive stroke.

Around the clock nurses came and went, caring for her deteriorating body. When the nurses weren't present, family members assisted with her care. Because there was almost no fat remaining on her frail body, we had to be very careful to protect her from injury when changing her position in bed.

We roamed in and out of the room behind the nurses. We gave each other supportive hugs, laughed and cried about the good times, and showered my sister with love. Looking back, I think we all knew that we were saying our final goodbyes to her.

If you've ever watched a loved one suffer, you can understand what I mean when I say, *"It's a powerless feeling."* It was one of the times that I wished I wasn't a professional nurse, for I knew too well my sister couldn't sustain life in her condition.

Even more difficult, this was déjà vu for me. I was losing another beloved sibling to a preventable disease. My oldest brother died from complications of hypertension at age fifty-one, and my youngest brother died of AIDS at age thirty-five. My only surviving brother, now fifty-seven, has had two heart attacks, one when he was in his forties. And both my parents died from cardiovascular diseases. My large family of nine members had prematurely dwindled down to four.

Imagine the fear welling up inside of me while I cared for my ailing sister. I wanted to dash out of the room and regress back forty years to a time when my entire family was alive, my siblings and I had our whole lives ahead of us, and dying of disease was unfathomable in our young minds.

That experience alone made me deeply concerned about African American children who must watch their relatives suffer from debilitating illnesses and die young. They look at the quality of life of their ailing mothers, fathers, grandparents, aunts and uncles, and lose hope for their own futures. In addition, they hear of many African American celebrities and entertainers such as Barry White, age 58; Nell Carter, age 54; Rick James, age 56; Luther Vandross, age 54; and Gerald Lavert, age 40, who become ill or die much too young from preventable diseases.

We often hear our community leaders talk about how African American youth need to "stop the violence" because they are dying too young from gang wars and drugs. The irony is that although the leaders preach the importance of stopping the violence and the killing, they fail to show the next generation how to value quality of life when they do not manage their own health.

PAST BEHAVIOR + PRESENT BEHAVIOR = FUTURE BEHAVIOR

Children adopt behaviors from those who raise and lead them. Our health is in such poor shape that some of us are "walking time bombs" waiting to explode. I honestly fear that if we continue to lack consciousness about the importance of maintaining quality health, *we will soon be an extinct people.* This may sound extreme, yet the statistics I will cite later indicate that my concerns are well founded.

My family's health history, similar to other African American families, is part of a disastrous trend that has become much too common. I'm disheartened and disappointed by this fact.

A big part of my disappointment is that my family didn't consider *quality* of life over *quantity.* Does this mean that I believe that had they considered quality of life they would still be around today? Not necessarily.

But I do believe that caring for your health is not just about living longer—it is also about having optimum health as well. *Optimum health* means less illness, less health concerns, more energy and vitality at every age.

One of the best ways to ensure optimum health is by keeping your immune system strong. The immune system is your body's natural defense against infections, viruses, toxins, and parasites that try to invade your body. When your immune system is strong it can fight invasions and diseases with greater rigor. Studies suggest that good nutrition, stress reduction, and regular exercise are effective in strengthening the immune system. You may still get sick, you may even have a major health problem, but if a health challenge occurs, your body will handle it better if your immune system is working effectively.

It is imperative that we, as African Americans, stop being casual about our health. When we neglect our health there are serious consequences that affect not only us as individuals, but also extend to our families and our communities.

My personal prayer is that through the pages of this book you will be a little more enlightened about your own health and wellness, and a lot more motivated to try new ways to improve it.

When you are concerned about your health and seek ways to improve it—*you're taking the quality of your life into your own hands.*

CHAPTER 3

Blacks "Do" Crack

"Blacks don't crack." If you've never heard this old adage, it may be because it outdates you. It is an ancient saying among African Americans referring to the fact that people of African descent have a great advantage over other races—we scarcely wrinkle because of the abundance of *melanin* in black skin.

Melanin is the chemical substance that primarily determines human skin color. It is the darkness of skin, hair, or eyes resulting from a high degree of pigmentation. Melanin, which absorbs ultraviolet light, plays a protective role when skin is exposed to the damaging rays of the sun. Because of this, our black skin shows minimum signs of lines, folds, and wrinkles as we age.

So, the saying that blacks don't crack has merit and is an extra benefit for being born of African descent.

Many African Americans, however, misinterpret "blacks don't crack" as meaning that their entire body, external and internal, will not give way with age.

Take my mother, who was a beautiful chocolate-skinned woman. She was seventy years old when she passed, but her skin had remained silky smooth and wrinkle free. If you looked at her skin, you could not detect that she had suffered numerous strokes, plus had heart problems that ultimately took years off her life. My point is that although blacks may not crack on the outside, *Blacks "Do" Crack on the inside.*

When it comes to disease and illness, we frequently hear dire reports about the African American state of health. *"African Americans are dying at higher rates of this, or a higher rate of that,"* the media proclaims.

Sometimes I doubt the validity of these reports, or try my best to tune them out. But the sad reality is that they are based on factual data.

As much as I dislike hearing these statistics, I dread having to remind you of them. Here are the dreaded facts:

- *African American men's* **life expectancy** *is 69.8 years compared to 75.7 years for white men. African American women's* **life expectancy** *is 76.5 years compared to 80.8 years for white women.*
- *African Americans are 30 percent more likely to die of* **heart disease** *than whites.*

- *One out of three African Americans suffer from **high blood pressure**, which is the number one risk factor for stroke.*

- *45 percent of African American men and 46 percent of African American women have total blood **cholesterol** levels that are above the acceptable level of 200 mg/dL.*

- *African American adult onset of **diabetes** is 70 percent higher than white Americans, and we are more likely to develop diabetic complications including kidney disease, blindness, and amputations.*

- *African American women are more than twice as likely to die of **cervical cancer** or **breast cancer** than any other ethnic group. And African American men have the highest rate of **prostate cancer** and death in the world, as well as die more often from **cancer of the lung** than do white men.*

- *For **all types of cancer**, and at **all stages**, African Americans have a decreased likelihood of survival five years after diagnosis than other ethnic groups.*

- *61.7 percent of African American men twenty years and older are **overweight**, and 28.9 percent are **obese**. 77.7 percent of African American women twenty years and older are overweight, and 50.4 percent are obese.*

These are *just a few* of the bleak facts about the present state of African American health. Disheartening isn't it? And worse, many of the African Americans who do manage to live into old age have *poor quality health.*

Although these statistics are factual, what mainstream media too often fails to share with the general public are the important factors that contribute to the health disparities between African Americans and other ethnic groups.

Referring to these racial/ethnic health disparities, the Centers for Disease Control and Prevention (CDC) reports, "For blacks in the United States, health disparities can mean earlier deaths, decreased quality of life, loss of economic opportunities, and perceptions of injustice." The CDC further reports, "Factors contributing to poor health outcomes among African Americans include discrimination, cultural barriers, and lack of access to health care."

Let's consider **lack of access to health care,** which is a concern that has spread well beyond the African American community. Many African Americans do not have health insurance and cannot afford preventive health care. This is partly due to a high unemployment rate among African Americans, which translates to a large population of people who are not afforded health coverage through work benefits. And for those African Americans who are employed, the high cost of health insurance premiums make health care unaffordable. This results in low-income patients experiencing difficulties or delays accessing health care.

Racism in the health care system is the root cause of many statistical disparities when comparing African Americans' health to white Americans' health. It should not be a surprise when I say African Americans do not receive the same quality of health care as white Americans. Studies have shown that despite advances in the modern medical system, racial and ethnic minorities still receive less care and/or lower-quality care than white Americans.

This message was reinforced when former Surgeon General David Satcher, MD, presented startling data on the issue of racial and ethnic disparities in 2002. He referred to the Institute of Medicine's (IOM) report "Unequal Treatment," which found that minorities receive lower-quality health care than whites even when insurance status, income, age, and severity of illness are comparable. The report also emphasized that differences in treating heart disease, cancer and HIV infection partly contribute to higher death rates among minority groups.

Distrust in the health care system also contributes to racial health disparities. Specific events, such as the Tuskegee Syphilis Experiment, do little to reduce the mistrust. For forty years between 1932 and 1972, the U.S. Public Health Service (PHS) conducted an experiment in Macon County, Alabama on 399 black men who were in the late stages of syphilis. The men were never told what disease they had. They were told only that they were being treated for "bad blood." The purpose of the experiment was to discover how syphilis affected blacks as compared to whites. The data for the study was to be collected from the men's autopsies. The black men were deliberately denied treatment, even though penicillin was discovered as a treatment in the 1940's. Memory of this and other atrocities still lingers in the minds of many older African Americans. As a result, African Americans delay or avoid seeking medical attention, further debilitating their health.

Access to healthy food is one of the greatest concerns I have when considering racial health disparities. I have lived in a predominately African American community for many years and I can personally attest to the limited access we have to quality foods. I'm forced to drive twelve miles from my home to buy organic produce and other healthy food items that I can't find in my own community.

According to a study of 261 food markets in Los Angeles done by the African Americans Building a Legacy of Health Coalition/REACH 2010 Project, stores in low-income areas had half the variety of fruits and vegetables as stores in the more affluent west side communities of Los Angeles. In addition, fruits and vegetables in many stores in low-income areas were damaged or dirty.

A study conducted by the University of North Carolina found that in many predominantly black neighborhoods poor eating habits may stem from a lack of fresh, nutritious food, noting that produce consumption *increased* 32 percent for each additional supermarket. This means that if African Americans in low-income communities had access to healthier foods, they would likely consume them. The study involved 208 neighborhoods in Maryland, North Carolina, Mississippi, and Minnesota.

In addition to the lack of fresh, nutritious foods, many low-income neighborhoods have **more fast food restaurants** than grocery chains or fine dining facilities. This means that people in lower-income communities have more access to artery-clogging fried chicken, hamburgers, and French fries than they do fresh fruits and vegetables.

It is amazing how many fast food chains have sprung up on every corner within a two-mile radius of my home. There are (4) McDonald's, (1) Burger King, (1) Church's Fried Chicken, (2) Taco Bell, (1) El Pollo Loco, (1) Carl's Jr. Burgers, (2) Louisiana Fried Chicken, (1) Jack in the Box, (2) Chinese fast food places, and numerous independent hamburger stands.

Changing the factors that cause health disparities for African Americans is a complex task that will take years to address. It will likely require changing government policy and laws, changing the American health care system, and changing the racial prejudices embedded in the minds of many—all of which are long-term goals that are not always in our immediate control.

So what is in our control? What personal responsibility can we take to close the gap of health disparities between us and other ethnic groups? Maybe we don't have direct control over the socioeconomic factors that impact our communities, but we do have the power to effect change in our own lives by *making healthier lifestyle choices.*

This is the only way that we can remain as preserved on the inside as our beautiful smooth skin is on the outside.

CHAPTER 4

Acceptance/Denial

Being a health care professional, I frequently talk about health with people from all walks of life. The conversations that impact me the most are those I've had with my own people, people of African American descent.

I started keeping a journal of comments made by my people regarding health. Sometimes I was so shaken by the prevailing thoughts sweeping through the community about health that I didn't have to take notes: I couldn't forget the comments if I tried, because the people speaking were suffering from major illnesses such as cancer, diabetes, hypertension, or heart disease.

Most disturbing was the lack of acceptance and outright denial of responsibility in the attitudes of those speaking about their health. Over and over I heard statements such as:

"This is something that God put on me."
"There's nothing I can do to change it now."
"What I don't know won't hurt me."
"If it don't kill me, it'll make me fat."
"I can't help it, it 'runs' in my family."
"I don't claim it" or "I don't receive it."
"A little bit won't hurt me."

I have heard it all. But even though I've heard these clichés and expressions all my life, I began to listen with new understanding. People were expressing a lack of control over their health. By this I mean that they disassociated themselves from the consequences of their behavior — classic cases of denial.

CASE IN POINT

"I Have To Die From Something"

I was having lunch with a young lady one day, who was eating a burrito she'd bought from someone selling food door-to-door in her neighborhood. When I asked her what was in the burrito, she answered, "Some kind of meat. I don't know what it is but it really tastes good." The burrito was packaged without a label.

I suggested that she be cautious about eating packaged foods without labels because they may contain something that could make her sick. She replied, *"What's the big deal? I have to die from something."*

I agree that we have to die from *something*, but do we have to be suicidal about it? I don't doubt that this young lady's burrito tasted good, even delicious, but what was she eating? Dog meat? Rat meat? Or was it meat at all?

Because something tastes good does not mean it's good for you! You should always know what you are eating, and care about how it could affect your health.

Take a few seconds to read the food labels that list ingredients. The U.S. Food and Drug Administration (FDA) established food labels to make it easier for you to make informed, healthier choices when shopping, comparing foods, and planning healthy meals.

The nutrition food label provides you with information that includes expiration dates to prevent you from eating food that is not safe for consumption, and a list of the ingredients in the food, including food additives.

If there isn't a label, inquire about the food's content. If you can't get a straight answer, don't eat it! *It won't kill you not to eat it… but it may if you do.*

Think about it. Does it make good health sense not to know what you are eating and how it could affect you? The answer is no. However, there are people who actually are aware of the negative effects that certain foods have on them, yet continue to consume these foods knowing they will suffer afterwards.

CASE IN POINT

"I Love To Eat"

Dela is a 50-year-old woman who jokingly refers to herself as "a human garbage can." She loves to cook, eat, and talk about food. When it comes to food preferences, as long as it is juicy and fat, she's satisfied. Most of her life she suffered from painful boils (pus-filled knots on the skin). She was destined to have boils, she said, because they "run in my family." Sometimes the infected boils would grow as big as golf balls in her groin area, under her arms, under her breast, on her back, and face. Periodically these boils would have to be surgically opened and drained. The boils often would get infected and she would have to take antibiotics.

Eventually she sought out an alternative health practitioner. The practitioner prescribed a diet consisting of fish, vegetables, brown rice, whole grains and limited fruits, and eliminated all red meat, chicken, processed foods, and sugar. And, she was given herbs to detoxify (clean out) her digestive system. In a few months she was free of boils and felt better than she had for years.

Unfortunately, because of Dela's "love" for fat greasy food, she relapsed to her old ways of eating. Subsequently the boils returned.

When you have this kind of attachment to food, it could mean that you are satisfying an *emotional need* rather than a nutritional one. In other words, you are "in love" with food versus simply loving food.

We are emotional beings and may not always make rational choices. As with some love relationships, it doesn't matter how detrimental the relationship is, or how bad you are being treated, you can love the person so much that you will try almost anything to make it work.

The same goes for when you are "in love" with food. You know that some foods are not good for you, but you eat them anyway. They can run up your blood pressure and your blood sugar, destroy your kidneys, damage your heart, keep your stomach so upset that you cannot sleep at night, give you splitting headaches, and make you so obese that your knees and back give out—but you don't mind because *you love the taste of the food!*

To a point it's okay to love food. Food is a necessity and often a pleasure to eat. It's the color of food that fascinates me. I love to sit down to a plate of green leafy vegetables, contrasted by bright orange carrots, or red juicy strawberries surrounded by green grapes and melons.

So I'm not faulting those who love food. Yet, a relationship with food, like any other "love affair," should be a healthy relationship that nourishes you emotionally, physically, and spiritually. If the relationship is toxic and results in ailments, *then it's not good for you.*

Warning signs may appear early in a relationship, but we ignore them and keep the relationship going. Over time we began to blame the other person for how they make us feel. What we don't do is take personal responsibility for our contribution to the problem.

In a similar way, when we have a poor relationship with food that makes us feel bad or ill, we sometimes blame God for "putting it" (as in the disease) on us. We refuse to acknowledge the illness, or take responsibility for our part in its development.

CASE IN POINT

"I Don't Claim It"

Joe is 48 years old. As a professional engineer and religious man, he takes pride in caring for his family and his job. But when it comes to his health, Joe is neglectful. He refuses to accept that he has Type II diabetes. *"I don't claim it,"* Joe said when he learned of his diagnosis. This is a common expression used by African Americans.

Joe's doctor informed him that his diabetes was mild and could be controlled with diet and exercise. But Joe chose not to follow the doctor's treatment plan. He continued to eat foods high in sugar and starch, and did not exercise. His blood sugar levels stayed so high, he was eventually prescribed oral medications. Again, Joe was noncompliant.

With Joe's diabetes now out of control, the doctor had to prescribe insulin injections. Again, Joe's response was "I don't claim it." He administered the injections a couple of times and then stopped.

By refusing to take his condition seriously and not following his doctor's prescribed treatment, Joe developed hypertension, heart disease, and eventually was put on dialysis treatments for kidney failure.

Years ago I had a very frightening experience when I discovered a lump in my right breast. My first fear was cancer. I knew there was a possibility that I could lose a breast, or even worse, die. I was very scared. Like Joe I did not want to "claim it." I wanted to ignore it as if the problem was not there. But I knew deep down inside that the best thing for me to do was to have a medical examination.

It took a while for me to get an appointment because the public health facility had a long waiting list. In the meantime, I prayed. When I finally got an appointment, the doctor confirmed there was a suspicious lump in my breast, and that I needed to have it removed. This occurred before lumpectomies (removal of lumps from the breast) were treatment options. Back then doctors would routinely perform a mastectomy (removal of the entire breast). While I waited for my scheduled surgery, I continued to pray.

One day while watching television, even though I did not know it at the time, my prayer was being answered. A doctor by the name of Bernie Siegel was being interviewed. He is one of the world's foremost physicians, authors, motivational speakers, and advocates for individuals facing the challenges of chronic illnesses. He is also a cancer survivor who helps others become aware of their own healing power.

I was particularly interested in his discussion about "creative visualization," which is a technique of using your imagination to create what you want in life. Using your mind, you create a clear image of something you wish to manifest. Then you continue to focus on the idea or picture regularly, giving it positive energy until it becomes an objective reality. Dr. Siegel taught cancer patients to use their minds to imagine their cancer cells being eaten away by some object, like Pac-Man.

Andrew Weils, M.D., in his book *Health and Healing*, also talked about the use of visualization. He described how a man rid himself of a ganglion cyst in two months by visualizing a white light going through it.

I had a really good feeling about this technique, so after doing more research on the subject, I decided to give it a try. Throughout the day I would picture in my mind an image of the lump in my breast and see it dissolve away.

I checked into the hospital the night before my scheduled surgery. The next morning the nurses prepared me for surgery, and I was given medication to help me to relax. A group of doctors making their rounds came into my room. One of them checked my breast, but could not find the lump. Then another doctor stepped up and he too did not find the lump. The lump had apparently dissolved. I was subsequently discharge from the hospital.

Some may call this miraculous, and perhaps it was. However, had I not "claimed" the problem, and had I not been proactive about getting it taken care of, perhaps none of the circumstances that led to my healing would have occurred.

For those individuals like Joe who have a religious foundation, my question to you is this: *How can God heal something that does not exist?* When you accept health challenges, you open channels to receive divine intervention.

However, if you remain in a state of denial, the disease can fester in your body and can progress to a stage where you will become very sick, disabled, or die.

ACCEPTANCE + PRAYER + HEALTH CARE = HEALING

Charles Swindoll

"The longer I live, the more I realize the impact of attitude on my life. Attitude to me is more important than facts, more important than the past, than education, than money, than circumstances, than failures, than successes, than what other people think or say or do... It is more important than appearance, giftedness or skill. It will make or break a company...a church...a home.
The remarkable thing is we have a choice every day regarding the attitude we will embrace for the day. We cannot change our past. We cannot change the fact that people will act in a certain way. We cannot change the inevitable. The only thing we can do is play on the string we have, and that is our attitude. I am convinced that life is 10% of what happens to me, and 90% of how I react to it. And so it is with you...
We are in charge of our attitudes."

CHAPTER 5

Attitude Shapes Behavior

Many of the diseases and illnesses that cause death and disability among African Americans are either curable, or can be greatly improved with proper nutrition and exercise. So why do so many African Americans have poor eating habits, lack commitment to exercise, and haphazardly manage their medical conditions? I say we need an *attitude adjustment*, as Charles Swindoll so eloquently said in the previous quotation.

Our attitude is the way we think, feel, or act that shows our disposition or opinion about something. **Attitude shapes behavior**. Whatever attitudes we have, good or bad, will affect how we feel about it, and determine our response to it. But, the attitudes that shape our behavior do not simply happen. They are learned, and generally come from perceptions we had earlier in life.

Historically, the negative images and oppressive conditions that we, as African Americans, have been subjected to, clearly indicate that our lives have not been valued in America. The devaluing of African American life continues to be perpetuated in the health care system, the criminal justice system, and American society in general. Over time, many of us have internalized this negativity, which manifests in low self-esteem.

Our attitudes have a lot to do with our self-esteem. Self-esteem is judgment of self worth as it relates to belief in oneself, and respect for oneself. Positive self-esteem is important for our overall health and wellness as human beings. On the other hand, poor self-esteem can create anxiety, stress, and increase vulnerability to overeating, as well as drug and alcohol abuse.

Whatever attitudes and beliefs we have about ourselves ultimately affect what we do and the decisions that we make, regardless of who we are or what our chosen professions might be.

CASE IN POINT

"The Health Committee"

The Health Committee is a group of professionals whose purpose is to develop programs and strategies to help African Americans improve their health. The group, which is composed primarily of African Americans, includes physicians, nurses, nutritionists, psychologists, social workers, and leaders from various community organizations. Some of the committee members themselves suffer from chronic diseases such as diabetes, high blood pressure, heart disease, and several of them are morbidly obese.

During the Health Committee meetings, food is served. If it's a breakfast meeting, the foods are generally high in sugar and fat, including donuts, coffee cakes, concentrated fruit juices, fruit yogurts, coffee with cream and sugar. Fresh fruits are sometimes available, but rarely eaten. If it's a lunch meeting, it is usually fatty foods high in sodium and sugar, such as fried chicken, potato salad, bread, soda, chips and dips, and sugary desserts. Raw vegetables are sometimes available but rarely eaten.

The paradox in this case is that the members of the Health Committee consistently stuff themselves with foods that are known to cause heart disease, diabetes, hypertension, and obesity *while they are developing programs to educate their clients about how to maintain health and prevent illnesses.* How can health professionals be so indifferent to what affects their own health? It seems that they have a total disconnect from their own bodies, as if their minds live a separate life.

Am I picking on health professionals? Yes, I am. It is one of my biggest pet peeves about the health care industry. My intention is to show how many health professionals have the same destructive attitudes regarding health as African Americans in other walks of life, regardless of their knowledge.

As a health professional myself, I feel that my attitude toward my own health has an impact on those I come in contact with. Generally, people look to health care professionals for guidance. We are the examples, or should be, for others to follow.

Also, I feel that health professionals have a great responsibility to assist in the health and well being of our community. However, we can only do this by raising our personal level of consciousness and moving beyond our own negative health attitudes. We can do this by developing a new mindset of how we view ourselves in relation to the people we serve.

This involves:

- Being healthy role models for others: *We cannot expect our clients to do something that we don't do.*
- Realizing that we are also a part of the community that we serve: *When we are not healthy, the community is not healthy.*
- Taking charge of our own health: *If we don't, we will not be around to take care of others.*

Although African Americans have been able to overcome many adversities in a racist society, we still struggle with the negative attitudes and perceptions that we have about ourselves. It is said that if you think something long enough you will start to believe it.

When you have a negative attitude about yourself, consciously or subconsciously, you are not likely to value your life as something that is precious and deserving of care. As such, circumstances relevant to quality of life and healthy life choices probably will not be at the top of your priority list.

Conversely, when you think of your life as valuable, and feel that as a human being you are worthy of the best, you are more likely to make healthier lifestyle choices.

Saying positive affirmations daily can help change the negative attitudes you may have about your health, and move you in a new healthier direction. Positive affirmations are statements you say to yourself that counteracts negative thoughts and beliefs. Affirmations can be repeated throughout the day, silently or out loud. Post your affirmations in various locations around your house, such as on your refrigerator or mirror. Or, take time to write out your affirmations every morning or evening. To help you get started, here are some examples of positive affirmations:

Positive Affirmations

- I am confident in myself.
- I am worthy of being respected.
- I choose to be healthy, well, and love who I am.
- I love to care for my body and my body cares for me.
- I have the power to control my health and wellness in every aspect of my life.
- I make a conscious choice of eating healthy foods that nourish my body to keep it healthy.
- I give myself permission to rest and heal without guilt.
- I have developed a harmonious working relationship between my mind and my body.
- I consciously create a mental, emotional, and spiritual attitude of confidence, serenity, and peace.
- I know that all things are possible, and with God's grace I now create my own vibrant health through my thoughts, words, and actions.

Dennis O'Grady

*"High self-esteem
results from making
small positive changes
in spite of fear.
Confidence
comes from conquering
fear of change."*

CHAPTER 6

Times Have Changed

Old Times

Our culture influences our food habits and customs. Culture is a way of life of a particular society or a group of people that includes their beliefs, values, attitudes, and behavior. Culture is learned and passed down from generation to generation.

Many cultural and historical factors influence how the African American diet has evolved into what it is today. This is especially true as it relates to the deplorable period of slavery when blacks were not privileged to eat the same foods as their slave owners.

As such, slaves were given the scraps that were tossed out the back door by whites who considered the food garbage and not fit for human consumption. For example, parts of the pig such as hog maws (the pig's stomach), feet, ears, and chitlins, ("chitlins"), the intestines, and other discarded pig parts.

However, since slaves were allowed to have very little meat, if any, their diet was primarily vegetables, fruits, and grains that were rich in vitamins and minerals. The vegetables were the discarded tops of turnips, beets, dandelions, and weeds that were gathered from the fields and grown in gardens.

Eventually blacks were introduced to other types of greens such as collard, kale, mustard, and spinach. Many of the hearty nutritious foods such as grains, legumes, yams, watermelon, okra, and leafy greens, were already indigenous to the African continent.

According to research, some slaves actually ate better than their owners who consumed mostly fatty foods, few vegetables, lots of sweets, and drank too much alcohol.

Slaves were given meager weekly rations of corn meal, salt pork, flour, and molasses. They used these ingredients in various combinations to create a variety of tasty dishes. Leftover fish was used to prepare croquettes, and the nutritious liquid from cooked greens, called "pot likker," was used in gravies. Salt pork and lard added flavor to the cooked vegetables and soups.

Cornmeal was used to make bread, and for dessert they would mix the cornmeal with molasses. They also used stale bread to make a delicious dessert that has become a longtime favorite in American culture—bread pudding.

New Times

The traditional African American diet, and the style of cooking that was coined "soul food" in the 60's and 70's, is based in part on the food practices and customs handed down from the time of slavery.

When I think of soul food I see images of deep fried foods saturated with fat, mustard greens and red beans flavored with greasy animal fat, mashed potatoes swimming in butter, and macaroni layered with cheese. We have virtually eliminated the part of the slave diet that was rich in vegetables, fruits, and grains, and have maintained the part that is saturated with fat and grease.

Some of the same foods that were considered substandard during slavery, like chitlins, are now thought of as delicacies. As a matter of fact, it is traditional for many African Americans to celebrate "New Years" with a meal of hog headcheese, chitlins, macaroni and cheese, and load the otherwise nutritious black-eyed peas, cabbage, and greens with greasy "fat back." *Sound familiar?*

It is believed that this meal will bring you good luck in the New Year. How many people who eat this artery-clogging food at the beginning of the year will be "lucky" enough to be around to talk about it at the end of the year?

I can remember when my mother used to cook chitlins. The smell was so bad that we had to open all the windows in the house to stand it. It would take her hours to clean them, remove the fat, and the waste material (feces). She cooked them for hours and used an abundance of seasoning to kill the incredible stench. Personally, I never had a desire to cook chitlins. However, back then, I did like *eating* them smothered in hot sauce.

Of course, many cultures besides African American celebrate holidays and special events like weddings, family reunions, funerals, and graduations with food. During these celebratory times, people tend to indulge in richer and fattier foods than normal. Although people may get away with eating this way once or twice a year, many African Americans, even those who have "given up the pig," continue to eat this way on a day-to-day basis. The sad reality is that, as they continue to consume these foods, they are getting fatter, and sicker.

CASE IN POINT

"No Matter How Hard I Try, I Can't Lose Weight"

Margie is a 39-year-old morbidly obese woman who says that her weight problems began after she had children. She is always nibbling on something, and wants to taste everyone else's food. A typical breakfast for her is pancakes with syrup and butter, scrambled eggs, bacon, and coffee with cream and sugar. Lunch is fried chicken, French fries, bread, and soda. And dinner is smothered steak and gravy, macaroni and cheese, bread, canned string beans with salt pork, a lettuce salad with ranch dressing, and some type of sugary dessert.

Though she doesn't exercise, Margie cannot understand why she is unable to lose weight after trying every imaginable diet. "They just do not work!" she claims.

As a result of her obesity, Margie has developed high blood pressure, and has torn ligaments in her knees. She has difficulty walking, and her doctor said she will need knee surgery to correct the problem.

When you consistently eat large portions of foods, and claim that you don't understand why you can't lose weight, you are in deep denial. "Closet eaters" epitomize such denial. They may tell others "*I don't eat that much,*" when in reality they are eating beyond much. What closet eaters don't realize is that their appearance gives them away. In other words, if you look like you eat too much—then you probably eat too much.

The undeniable fact is that if you eat less, and exercise more, you will not gain weight—you will lose it. If you do not believe me you should visit a third world country where people are deprived of food. I'm certain that you won't find many who are overweight.

We must keep in mind that during slavery blacks did not live a sedentary lifestyle like African Americans do today. Slaves spent many hours laboring in the fields and burned off the high amount of fat in their diets.

It is also important to realize that, in general, eating in America has changed tremendously. Food eaten today is vastly different than prior decades when people did not eat "fast food" or consume processed foods that might taste good but have little or no nutritional value.

Years ago fruits and vegetables were grown on local farms, not imported from other parts of the world. People ate more whole grains, legumes, nuts, and seeds. The crops were not laced with chemical pesticides and fertilizers that deplete the food of its nutritional value and expose you to health problems like cancer.

The meats came from healthy animals that were not injected with hormones. Hormones are used to accelerate the growth rate of animals so that they can reach market earlier. Overuse of hormones has been linked with the escalating incidence of cancer, and many other health problems in humans.

The antibiotics administered to chickens, cows, pigs, and other livestock, contribute to the development of antibiotic-resistant infections in humans.

When I was growing up in Los Angeles, we raised our own chickens. Our chickens were corn fed and hormone free. My dad would go out to the chicken coup early Sunday morning and select a chicken for dinner. It seems cruel to me now but he would hold the chicken by its neck and wring it until it snapped. Then my mother would remove the feathers from the chicken, clean and cook it.

Chickens and their eggs tasted and smelled totally different from the common foul odor that they have today; an odor that can only be masked if deep fried, barbequed, baked or smothered with lots of seasoning.

When you consider how processing food depletes it of many nutrients, and how we further destroy the value of foods through overcooking and added fats, it is clear that we are not getting what we need to maintain our health.

It is virtually impossible for the human body to sustain itself without adequate nutrition.

I am not suggesting that you give up all of your favorite foods, or abandon tradition. What I am suggesting is that you stop clinging to your old harmful habits and explore new, healthier ways of preparing the foods that you like. I'll give you many examples in Part II, such as specific spices and herbs to flavor vegetables instead of fatty meats.

You will discover that your diabetes, high blood pressure, and high cholesterol will start to normalize and may even disappear as you move away from the overuse of fats, sugars, and salts.

Lottie Mallory-Perkins

*"My body is my shelter
and every aspect of it
needs to be healthy
in order for me to have
a safe place to live."*

CHAPTER 7

Prevention Goes a Long Way

The most effective way to manage your health is through prevention, because it is much easier to maintain health and wellness than it is to regain your health after you become ill. It is not uncommon for people to make the mistake of waiting until a major health crisis happens before they get concerned about their health. Often, they get signals from their bodies telling them that something is wrong, such as frequent headaches, dizziness, indigestion, blurred vision, or pain. But many times these signals are ignored, or thought to be insignificant.

Dr. Andrew Weil, M.D., in his book *Health and Healing* says, "*Failure to notice and recognize disease at early stages is one of the main reasons for its severity and stubbornness. The earlier you notice a medical problem, the less work will be needed to correct it, to modify its course so that its peak will not be so high and its duration not so long. The farther into its course a disease proceeds before therapeutic measures are applied, the stronger the measures need to be and the smaller their chance of succeeding.*"

Dr. Weil continues, "*Unless you learn to notice and be bothered by the early, subtle stages of illness, you will lose your chances of managing your body through its changing cycles by simple means and will find yourself more and more dependent on outside practitioners and the costly interventions of modern hospital medicine.*"

Remember, what you don't know CAN hurt you.

CASE IN POINT

"Eddie"

At age 58, Eddie lives on fast foods, fried foods, and sweets. He rarely eats fruits, vegetables, or anything that contains fiber. He doesn't think of himself as an overeater because he only eats a small amount of food at a time, even though by the end of the day he has consumed quite a lot. He doesn't worry about his extra pounds because he has no major health problems like high blood pressure or diabetes.

Although Eddie has been having mild symptoms of upset stomach, abdominal discomfort, and periodic constipation, he attributes this to his age. He thought that as long as laxatives and antacids provided temporary relief, he would be okay. He had not had a medical examination for many years. Eventually he was forced to see a doctor because his symptoms began to worsen; he was experiencing diarrhea, nausea, and extreme fatigue.

The doctor informed him that he was severely anemic, and blood was found in his stool. Subsequent tests revealed that Eddie had colon cancer.

How many times have you heard the statement, *"He was perfectly healthy, and then all of a sudden he was gone"?* In some cases like Eddie's, health problems that appear to happen overnight actually take place over a long period of time. The longer a health problem goes untreated, the greater the chances are that it will affect other parts of your body. Unlike a house with rooms separated by solid walls, your body is not compartmentalized. It consists of complex systems that are interactive and dependent on each other.

Eddie ignored the symptoms he was experiencing. These symptoms were his body's signals telling him that something unusual was occurring. Perhaps if he was having regular medical examinations and routine laboratory work, his cancer may have been detected before it had the opportunity to spread. (It is recommended that African American men have a colon examination at age forty-five). And, had Eddie included more fiber-rich foods in his diet, they may have helped to prevent the colon cancer altogether. (A diet *low* in fiber has been linked to the incidence of colon cancer).

You probably know someone with a life-threatening illness who failed to manage his or her conditions. Many people who have high blood pressure continue to eat sodium-laden foods. Those with diabetes continue to eat foods packed with starch and sugar. Others with heart disease and cholesterol problems continue to eat starchy, high fat foods. And many people refuse to take their prescribed medication.

Tune up or break down

It is quite amazing that people can be negligent when it comes to taking care of their bodies, yet conscientious when it comes to taking care of their *cars*. If they hear an unusual noise (symptom) coming from their car, they're off to the mechanic to check it out. They're diligent about getting their cars serviced regularly, and use the best oils and gas to ensure everything will keep running smoothly.

Because their cars are important to them, owners are particular about keeping them shiny and clean so that the car will look its best, and they will look their best when they drive it. Some people make caring for their automobile a ritual of washing and waxing, polishing and tinkering.

These are the same people who wake up every morning to a cup of coffee and half-dozen donuts, not realizing that putting sugar in your body is like putting sugar in your gas tank. It will damage your motor!

Just like your car, your body needs regular tune-ups in order to operate effectively. And, just like your car's warning indicators alert you when there is a problem, your body will alert you with signals when something has gone wrong. For example, when your blood pressure is very high, it is a major warning of a possible stroke or heart attack.

You should be as mindful of your body's warning signals as you are with your automobile's warning lights. You can start by taking an active role in managing your health by being "proactive"—taking conscious preventative measures such as the following:

1. **Be knowledgeable about your medical problems**

   The more you know about your health condition the better you will be able to take care of it by making informed decisions as an active participant in your health care.

   Ask your health practitioner for written information that is relevant to your diagnosis. Do your own research by visiting the library, or the Internet.

2. **Have regular medical evaluations**

   Regular medical check-ups (every 1-2 years) can help determine many things about your health that may otherwise go undetected, and identify some diseases before symptoms occur.

3. **Watch and record your symptoms**

   Keeping a record is valuable information that can help your health practitioner more accurately assess your medical situation. For the most part, a great deal of your care is based on the facts that you report.

   Although everyone experiences some symptoms once in a while, it is the intensity and frequency that can indicate when it is not a normal condition. At the first sign of a health problem, make note of the symptoms. Record when, how long, how painful, etc. (See sample Record of Symptoms and Health Concerns at the end of this section.)

4. **Be knowledgeable about your medications**

   If you need medication, make sure you understand what it's for and take it as your doctor recommends. This includes the name of the medication, how long you have to use it, the reason you need it, how long it takes to work, how to take it (with food, or on an empty stomach, etc), and, possible side effects or other risks.

   The more you know about your medications and their importance to your health condition, the more likely you are to take them, and take them correctly.

5. **Be knowledgeable about your prescribed diet**

   If you have a certain medical condition, such as diabetes or high blood pressure, and you are on a special diet, *follow* it. You cannot expect your condition to remain stable if you are not compliant.

6. **Don't be afraid to explore alternative treatments**

   There may be times when your regular medical care just doesn't do what you want it to do, and alternative treatment is a better option. For example, you have seen several doctors and your headaches have not gotten any better. Maybe acupuncture can help. Or, despite rest, exercise, and muscle relaxants, your back still hurts. Maybe a chiropractor can help.

7. **Get enough sleep**

   It is important that you get sufficient sleep. When your body tells you it is tired, you should rest. When you are fatigued, your resistance is lowered to infection, and other illnesses. Getting sufficient sleep is an essential part of a healthy lifestyle.

8. **Don't smoke**

Smoking increases your chances of developing a stroke, heart disease, peripheral arterial disease, and several forms of cancer. Each year, approximately 45,000 African Americans die from a preventable smoking-related disease.

If you have trouble giving up smoking, there are smoking-cessation programs that can help.

9. **Don't overindulge in alcohol**

Alcohol-related illnesses and accidents are one of the leading causes of death among African Americans.

High consumption of alcohol can increase your risk for high blood pressure, stroke, heart disease, certain cancers, and cirrhosis of the liver, birth defects and death.

Alcohol also plays a major role in automobile accidents, domestic violence, and suicide.

To decrease your risk of developing serious alcohol-related illnesses and accidents, you have to drink smaller amounts of alcohol, drink less frequently, or not drink at all.

You have a personal responsibility to maintain your own health and manage any illness before it gets out of control. Your body is your temple—a gift from God. Be grateful and take care of this precious gift.

Sample

RECORD OF SYMPTOMS AND HEALTH CONCERNS

DATE	TIME	ACTIVITY	SYMPTOMS/CONCERNS
10/1/00	5:00 PM	Watching TV	Difficulty breathing
10/1/00	11:30 PM	Laying in bed	Mild chest pain
10/2/00	**7:00 AM**	Walking	Heart pounds
10/2/00	12:00 PM	Lunch	Indigestion
10/3/00	2:00 PM	Working on computer	Chest tightness
10/3/00	4:00 PM	Shopping	Short of breath
10/4/00	9:00 AM	Driving	Feel tired
10/4/00	5:00 PM	Dinner	Indigestion
10/4/00	8:45 PM	Laying in Bed	Mild chest pain
10/5/00	8:00 AM	Breakfast	Bloated
10/5/00	10:00 AM	Driving	Feel Tired

Author Unknown

*"I allow myself to relax into the presence of God
that dwells within me.
In my imagination,
I see this stream of living water flowing from a well
that dwells deep within my being.
As I relax, this Divine water fills up my body,
healing and restoring my cells to radiant health.
My emotions become calm and peaceful
as the living waters soothe me.
My mind is cleansed of limiting thoughts and beliefs by the
power of this radiant energy."*

CHAPTER 8

Relax and Reduce Stress

The devastating effects that stress can have on health are of particular importance to African Americans. Certain social conditions such as discrimination, educational inequality, blocked opportunities, and poverty are major stressors. Stress contributes to the high rate of hypertension among African Americans: A study at the Morehouse School of Medicine in 1999-2001 suggests links between racism and high blood pressure in African Americans.

Stress is how our bodies physically and emotionally respond to changes in our life. These changes can be positive such as a marriage or the birth of a child, or negative like losing your job or the death of a spouse. We live in a highly stressful environment. No one can escape it. Stress is a fact of life and it is doubtful that this will ever change.

When you are under stress there are many profound physiological changes going on inside your body. In the 1950's, physiologist Hans Selye described stress as *"the nonspecific response of the body to any demand made upon it."*

The instant you are faced with a perceived threat, or stressor, whether it's real or imagined, your brain automatically sends signals to the rest of your body that triggers a chain of physiological changes. These changes prepare your body for intense mental and physical activity, often called the "fight or flight response" because it prepares you to either face the danger, or run from it.

The physical reactions to stress are known to be the following:

- Increased release of adrenalin hormone
- Increased heart rate
- Increased blood pressure
- Increased blood sugar
- Increased rate of breathing
- Pupils dilate
- Increased muscle tension
- Increased perspiration
- You feel a rush of strength and energy
- Your body is tense, alert and ready for action.

If the stress response is triggered frequently, the temporary effects, like the rise in blood pressure, become constant. This often leads to serious problems such as hypertension, heart disease and/or stroke. Also, prolonged stress weakens your immune system and decreases its ability to fight disease and illnesses.

Sometimes it's difficult to recognize, and admit, that high stress levels are affecting your health. One of the key points to stress management is to learn to listen to your body. And, although everyone responds to stress differently, your body will give you one or more of these clues:

- Chest pain
- Shortness of breath
- Extreme fatigue
- Headaches
- Insomnia
- Digestive problems
- Anxiety or panic
- Stiff neck
- Nagging backache
- Sweaty palms
- Irritability
- Depression

Eating disorders are another indicator: Stress can have a tremendous effect on the way you eat. How many times have you heard people say they "eat anything in sight" when they're stressed out? It's usually because they obtain some measure of comfort from eating. It's "comfort food," especially when it's high in carbohydrates. But consistently eating large amounts of food to relieve stress can result in serious health problems, like obesity and diabetes.

The reverse can also be a result of overwhelming stress. Some people lose their appetite and stop eating. This can lead to health problems like anemia, low blood sugar, and anorexia.

It's clear that both overeating and under-eating due to unrelieved stressful situations can lead to serious trouble.

Be aware of the signs from your body of too much stress in your life. Choose healthy ways to reduce mental, physical, and emotional stress. It is important to learn healthy coping behaviors, like relaxation, if the origin of the stress is something that cannot be changed immediately, or is out of your control.

Relaxation

Most of us think we know what relaxation is, but we can be confused about its purpose, and how it works. The relaxation techniques used in stress management have specific step-by-step guidelines. Some techniques are used to achieve muscle relaxation, while others are used to reduce anxiety and emotional arousal. Overall, relaxation helps relieve your body and mind of tension, helps you to focus, and helps you to deal with things more calmly.

The term "relaxation" can mean different things to different people. Some people use unhealthy relaxation techniques for managing stress such as self-medication with alcohol, drugs, or smoking. These methods may appear to promote relaxation, but in reality chemicals put even more stress on the mind and body.

I have heard people say that they relax by drinking a cup of coffee. The caffeine in coffee is a *stimulant* to the nervous system, making your body work even *harder* to relax. Others say that they relax by reading the newspaper, listening to the radio, or watching television. These activities, especially when they involve disturbing news reports, stimulate thought and emotional reactions—the opposite of relaxation.

The primary goal of relaxation is to turn off the outside world so that the mind and body are at rest. Therefore, at some point in the day you need to give your body and mind a chance to **stop**, be **quiet**, and be **still**.

It is understandable if you think there's no time after taking care of your family, working, shopping, cooking, cleaning, etc. to sit twice a day for 20 minutes practicing relaxation techniques. I most certainly relate because I started practicing Transcendental Meditation many years ago when my children were small. I was a full-time student at the time, plus worked part time. I didn't know how to fit meditation into my busy schedule.

It was quite awkward for me at first. After experimenting with meditating different times of the day, I found that the most practical time for me was early in the morning before my family awoke, and somewhere between dinner and homework in the evening. Eventually my family began to appreciate the time that I took for relaxation, and learned not to disturb me. If someone called or came by, my children got used to saying that *"My mother is meditating and will get back to you in a short while."*

When my children were older, they learned to meditate as well, and we would have quiet time together. Including them in the simple relaxation technique of meditation helped all of us. It also gave my children an effective tool they could use for managing stress throughout their lives.

The benefit to remember is that taking control and creating a time to manage stress will help you stay mentally and physically healthy. Get in the habit of spending some time each day that's not filled with frenzied activity. Make some peaceful moments in each day and you'll begin to see more peaceful qualities in everything around you.

In the 1970's, Dr. Herbert Benson, a specialist in cardiovascular medicine at Harvard Medical School, studied how the body responded to certain practices—Christian prayer, Transcendental Meditation (T.M.), biofeedback, hypnosis, and relaxation techniques called autogenic therapy and progressive relaxation. He discovered that the body showed a common response to all these techniques, which he called the "Relaxation Response." It consisted of lowering the heart rate, blood pressure, and breathing rate; reduced need for oxygen; less carbon dioxide production and so on. Benson found that although our intellects may differentiate between prayer and meditation, our bodies do not.

As noted in the above study, there are many types of relaxation techniques, and many books you can read about each one. Please explore the options and find one or more that you can fit into your life. They include: meditation (many forms), prayer, yoga, progressive muscle relaxation, visualization, imagination, biofeedback, self-hypnosis, and guided imagery.

Since I can't cover them all, I'll focus on my three favorites: *meditation, progressive muscle relaxation,* and *prayer.*

Don't be discouraged if it takes a little time for you to become accustomed to a new technique or exercise. Once you have trained your body and mind to relax, in perhaps three to four weeks, you'll be able to produce the same relaxed state whenever you desire to reduce tension and stress throughout the day.

Meditation

Meditation is a relaxation exercise that involves sitting quietly and focusing on your breathing, a word, or a sound—sometimes referred to as a "mantra." It is one of the most effective methods used to obtain deep relaxation.

In the unique meditative state of relaxation, your body functions differently than at any other time. Your metabolism is lowered, which means much less energy is expended, even less than during sleep.

It lowers the body's response to adrenaline and other hormones, including cortisol, the hormone associated with chronic stress.

Meditation has been used successfully in the prevention and treatment of high blood pressure, heart disease, and stroke. Its effects continue for many hours after the brief period of relaxation is accomplished.

Meditation Exercise

1. Find a quiet place where you can do the technique free from interruption or outside stimulation. It can be at home, where you work, or sitting in your car.
2. Adopt an attitude that this is your time. There are 24 hours in a day and you deserve at least 20 minutes of that time for yourself.
3. Get into a comfortable sitting position before you begin, shifting around until your body is at ease.
4. Close your eyes and focus your attention on your breathing. Take a few deep breaths in and then out through the nose. Let your breathing be slow and relaxed as you imag-

ine God's healing energy flowing through your body.

5. Now, as you inhale say "re" to yourself, and as you exhale say "lax." Draw out the pronunciation of the word so that it lasts for the entire breath. The "re" sounds like r-r-r-e-e-e-e-, and "lax" sounds like l-l-l-a-a-a-x-x-x. Repeating the word as you breathe will help you to focus.

6. Don't worry about your thoughts; just let them fade in and out of your mind freely. Become passive and detached from the thinking process.

7. Continue repeating step number 5 as you feel yourself falling deeper and deeper into relaxation, your body sinking into the chair.

8. After about 20 minutes, gradually stop saying the word "relax," and focus again on your breathing.

9. Take a few deep breaths through the nose. Let your breathing be slow and relaxed.

10. Remain sitting with your eyes closed for 1-2 more minutes. Take another deep breath and slowly open your eyes.

11. Practice this easy meditation exercise 20 minutes in the morning and 20 minutes in the evening.

Progressive muscle relaxation

Muscle relaxation is one of the most commonly used relaxation techniques. It is effective in combating stress and often helps people get to sleep. It's popular because it is easy to learn, and can be practiced in different situations at different times of the day.

To relax muscles, first you need to mentally scan your body to determine where you are holding tension. You'll probably find that you have areas where you experience most of your tension, such as the neck, shoulders, thighs, etc. It is precisely these areas that you want to repeatedly tense and relax. However, if you feel pain, tense those muscles very gently, or not at all, and focus instead on relaxation alone.

The following exercise will guide you to tense and then relax the major muscle groups in your body. Tense each muscle area for 5-10 seconds. Then give yourself 10-15 seconds to release it and relax.

Progressive Muscle Relaxation Exercise

1. Get in a comfortable position. Uncross your legs and ankles. Loosen any clothing that might feel tight.
2. Close your eyes and focus your attention on your breathing. Take a few deep breaths in and then out through the nose. Let your breathing be slow and relaxed.
3. Become aware of the muscles in your feet and calves. Curl your toes tight, and then slowly relax them.
4. Now tighten your thighs and buttocks. Hold and feel the tension, and then slowly relax them.
5. Take another deep breath, feeling yourself become more and more relaxed.
6. Tense the muscles in your abdomen and chest, and then slowly relax them.
7. Stretch your fingers out straight, tense your fingers and tighten your arm muscles, then slowly relax them.
8. Press your shoulder blades together, tightened the muscles in your shoulders and neck, and then slowly relax them.
9. Tighten the muscles in your face and head, wrinkling the forehead into a deep frown, and then release.
10. Now take another deep breath, stay still for a few more minutes, and enjoy the wonderful feeling of relaxation.
11. You can practice this relaxation technique at different times of the day.

Spirituality/Prayer

Having a source of inner peace and tranquility that fits your spiritual beliefs can make a tremendous difference in how you cope with stress.

The church has always been an intrinsic part of the African American community. Throughout all the struggles—slavery, the Civil Rights movement, right up to the challenges of today—the church has always been a source of hope, strength, and support. As such, many African Americans find comfort in prayer.

Modern research shows that prayer can have a positive influence on a number of health problems, and improve the likelihood of recovery from illness. For example, a study on cardiac patients, by Duke University and Durham Veterans Affairs Medical Centers, found that combining prayer with traditional treatments contributed to better outcomes. Other studies have found that people suffering from cancer, high blood pressure, and other ailments often improve the quality of their life with prayer.

Prayer is similar to meditation in that it helps to relax your body, create a positive environment, and relieve stress and tension. It has been said that prayer is when you talk to God, and that meditation is when you listen to what God has to say.

Other practical ways of managing stress

- Exercise regularly
- Eliminate or reduce sugar in your diet
- Eliminate or reduce caffeine
- Eliminate or reduce alcohol

- Don't smoke anything
- Get plenty of rest
- Get out into nature/get some sun
- Take a vacation
- Nurture yourself/take time for yourself
- Simplify your life
- Set realistic goals
- Talk over problems with family or a friend
- Learn an interesting hobby/skill
- Have more fun
- Get a massage or soak in a hot bath
- Don't be afraid to cry
- Learn how to forgive
- Don't dwell on the negative
- Laugh more often
- Do things you love, and love things you do
- Seek professional help when you are unable to cope.

Sample

RELAXATION EXPERIENCE

Take a moment to write down your relaxation experience. For example, *How does my body feel after performing the relaxation technique? Is there tension left anywhere?*

DATE	DESCRIPTION OF EXPERIENCE
1/1/00	I have less tension in my neck and shoulders.
1/2/00	I felt more relaxed and calm during the day.
1/3/00	I was able to fall asleep more easily then I normally do.
1/4/00	Overall, I have a greater sense of well being.

Henry Ford

*"Obstacles
are those frightful things
you see
when you take your eyes
off your goal."*

CHAPTER 9

Let Your Body Move

Lack of physical activity and exercise is unfortunately too much the norm for African Americans. Forty-six percent of African American men and fifty-seven percent of African American women are sedentary, with no time scheduled for exercise.

Physical inactivity increases the risk of many chronic illnesses such as diabetes, obesity, cardiovascular disease, and some types of cancer. One of the first things your doctor will advise, according to your ability, is to start an exercise program.

I've heard many excuses why you don't exercise: *"I don't need to exercise because I'm not overweight," "I don't have the time,"* or *"I get enough exercise when I work (or shop, or run after the kids)."*

However, the most prevalent justification I hear is, *"I just don't **like** to exercise."* Well, I don't **like** the statistics I've been quoting about illness and disease, so I will take this opportunity to remind you why you should do some form of exercise.

As a rule, people who exercise regularly feel better mentally and physically, and maintain their potential for functional independence as they go through the aging process.

An active lifestyle can help everyone. You don't have to be as fit as a professional athlete to benefit from physical activity. The value of consistent physical activity — and you can make it fun — cannot be overstated!

Moderate exercise on a consistent basis can make a tremendous difference in your mental and physical health, including:

1. **Improving your health and decreasing the risk of major illness**
   Lower high blood pressure
   Improve efficiency of the heart and lungs
   Lower cholesterol levels
   Help your body to use blood sugar more efficiently
   Improve muscle strength and flexibility
   Improve digestion

2. **Improving well-being**
   More energy
   Less stress
   Improve your mood
   Improve quality of sleep
   Increase mental alertness

3. **Improving appearance**
    Control weight
    Tone muscles
    Increase self-confidence

Starting a regular exercise program will be one of the best lifestyle changes you can make. It was for me. I have been exercising regularly for many years now. At first I joined a gym and did group aerobics, stretching, and worked out on a variety of machines. Then I was introduced to yoga and I fell in love with it. I have practiced yoga for 28 years, and eventually added daily walking to my program. Exercise is a now a way of life for me; I enjoy it, and look forward to the daily burst of energy and vitality that I feel afterwards.

So, forget all of the excuses about why you don't exercise. Get up off that couch and get to it!

Healthy options for moving your tired, stiff body

1. **Consult with your doctor**
    Talk to you doctor before starting an exercise program, especially if you have pre-existing health problems, or have not exercised for a long time.

2. **Choose the type of exercise that you like**
    If you don't like an exercise program, you will likely lose motivation to continue doing it.

3. **Walking is considered one of the best choices**
    Walking is a wonderful exercise that can be done by almost anybody. Walking is easy, safe and inexpensive. Once you get accustomed to exercising reg-

ularly, you can decide whether to continue walking or choose another form of exercise.

4. **Start out slowly and take it easy**
   Your body needs time to adapt to a new exercise program, even walking. So increase your walking gradually. Begin with 15-minute sessions, 3-4 times a week. Gradually increase until you are walking at least 30 minutes a day, 5-6 times a week.

5. **Listen to your body**
   Pay attention to your body's signals. It is important not to over-exert yourself. Exercise should be done regularly and in moderation. If you are in pain, or get too exhausted, don't force your body to continue. Stop and rest, or call it a day.

6. **Choose the right time of day for you**
   Exercise at a time that works well with your schedule, and stick to it. It can be morning, afternoon, or evening.

7. **Keep a record of your exercise activities**
   Making note of your exercise activities allows you to keep tract of your progress. (See the Weekly Physical Activity Log at the end of this section.)

8. **Keep your eyes on the prize**
   Don't get discouraged. It can take awhile before you notice some of the changes and benefits from your exercise program. Be patient and have fun!

Suggested Exercise/Physical Activities

Walking	Yoga	Bike riding
Stretching	Dancing	Jumping rope
Aerobics	Jogging	Running
Treadmill	Swimming	Climbing stairs
Gardening		

Sample

WEEKLY PHYSICAL ACTIVITY LOG

WEEK OF: _____

DAY/TIME	PHYSICAL ACTIVITY	HOURS	MIN	HOW I FELT
Monday 5 PM	Walking	1		Energized
Tuesday Noon	Bike riding		15	A little tired
Wednesday 7:30 AM	Yoga class		15	Relaxed
Thursday 5:00 PM	Walking		45	Energized
Friday 4:00 PM	Walking	1		Good mood
Saturday Noon	Walking	1		Alert
Sunday	No exercise today			

Lottie Mallory-Perkins

"The final responsibility
for your state of wellness
and overall health
is YOURS."

PART II

LEARNING HOW TO
EAT TO LIVE

Eating to Live

For me, this is the most important part of the book, because nourishing food is the single most important factor when learning how to eat to live, and striving to achieve good health. Without it you will not be able to exercise or meditate or do any of the other lifestyle changes I suggested in the previous chapters. As a matter of fact, without nourishing foods you would not be able to maintain a heartbeat for long.

It may sound simplistic to say that a poor diet can cause major health problems, even death. But when you consider that there are trillions of living cells in your body, it makes sense that these cells need nutrients to repair, heal, and maintain your health. So, there is no doubt that nutritious food is the single most important factor in achieving good health.

Looking back in time, we find that people such as medicine men, root doctors, and yes, our grandmothers, had the wisdom to use common foods, plants, and herbs to treat the sick and cure disease.

Today, we are coming full circle. Modern science has linked our eating habits directly to many ailments and diseases ranging from diabetes to arthritis. Research has clearly demonstrated that what and how we eat has a profound affect on human growth, development, aging, and the ability to live a viable productive life. So, common expressions such as "you are what you eat" and "food is your best medicine" have a lot of validity.

I want to emphasize that changing the way that you eat does not mean giving up all of your favorite foods, or abandoning African American tradition. What it means is finding nutritional alternatives for modifying the amount of fat, sugar, and salt (sodium) in your foods; and changing from the common ways of frying, barbequing, and overcooking foods.

Let me be clear; African Americans are not the only people in America that are becoming ill and dying from poor food choices. Over the past several decades, the health of the people in America has declined tremendously. Many of the physical problems plaguing this country today can be directly attributed to unhealthy diet and lifestyle choices.

Many Americans are suffering from poor health because of the Standard American Diet, referred to as "SAD," which is high in unhealthy fats, sodium, sugar, processed foods, low in fiber, and complex carbohydrates.

For me, what is even sadder than the "SAD" diet is the fact that the United States has spent more money on cancer research than any country in the world, yet the Standard American Diet contributes to the very diseases that they are spending money to prevent.

According to a statement in the 2005 Dietary Guidelines for America, published by the Department of Health and Human Services and Department of Agriculture: *"More than 90 million Americans are affected by chronic diseases and conditions that compromise their quality of life and well-being. Overweight and obesity, which are risk factors for diabetes and other chronic diseases, are more common than ever before. To correct this problem, many Americans must make significant changes in their eating habits and lifestyles."*

I started recognizing the influence my diet had on my health when I was diagnosed with high cholesterol. My cholesterol level was above the normal range of 200. I was advised to cut back on foods that were high in saturated fats, which is found primarily in animal products. I knew the potential health problems that high cholesterol could cause, and I took this advice very seriously because of my family history.

I immediately cut eggs, butter, and fried foods out of my diet. In just a couple of months my cholesterol dropped to 160. Eventually I made the decision to eliminate all animal products from my diet. I have been a vegetarian now for fifteen years. There is no cholesterol in plant-based foods. (Cholesterol is discussed in chapter 16.)

After lowering my cholesterol, I have monitored my body's responses to other foods by writing down any reactions that I may have in a "Food Sensitivity/Reaction Journal." (See a sample journal page at the end of this section.) By doing this, I have become more aware of my body's warning signals when certain foods do not agree with me.

For example, I noticed that when I eat sugary foods, even those sweetened with concentrated fruit juice, it causes joint pain and muscle stiffness. By limiting my consumption of sugary foods, I have essentially eliminated the problem. (Studies have shown that there is a link between sugar and arthritis.)

I continue to eliminate foods that have any adverse effect on my health, replacing them with healthier alternatives. For example, I have mastered some great cookie recipes that use whole fruits such as dates as an alternative to refined sugar. (Sugars are discussed in chapter 14.)

I admit it's not always easy for me to eliminate the foods, and it takes more time for some diet changes than for others. For example, I have stopped drinking coffee many times.

Once a year I visit the *Optimum Health Institute* in San Diego to help maintain my health program. This is a wonderful program that teaches people a total approach to cleansing the mind and body. The body is cleansed through a live-raw food diet, lymphatic exercise, the consumption of wheatgrass juice, and colon therapy. Guests learn about the purpose and process of cleansing by taking classes that focus on digestion, elimination, relaxation, and spiritual healing.

I believe that if you know why food is important to your health and well being, it will help you make better food choices: "Knowledge is Power." As Oprah says, *"If you know better, you will do better."*

I am not going to tell you that eating to live is going to be easy. Challenges like busy lifestyles, availability of fast food, persuasive advertising, and a lack of understanding of what healthy food is—all work against people who are trying to eat healthy. This I will discuss in detail as well.

But, what I will tell you is that your willingness to change poor health habits, whatever they are, will have a profound effect on the success and quality of your life.

Your mind and attitude can change in a minute, but your body needs time to adjust to changes, including exercise, meditation, and new ways of eating. _The key is not to try to change too much at once._ Instead, change one or two things at a time.

Remember you are developing healthy choices that will become a new, healthier *way of living*.

Therefore, it is important to acknowledge that you are an individual with your own particular set of needs. Your starting point for change, and your progress, will differ from anyone else's. However, if you suffer from an illness, I suggest that you start making changes as soon as possible, and always consult with your health care provider.

Now that you have accepted responsibility for your health, adjusted your attitude, gained understanding of the cultural influences of our food habits and customs, and learned how to manage your health through prevention, stress management, and exercise, you are prepared to learn how to EAT TO LIVE.

SAMPLE

FOOD SENSITIVITY/REACTION JOURNAL

DATE	TIME	FOOD/BEVERAGE	HOW DO I FEEL?
1/1/00	8:00 AM	3 pancakes syrup butter 2 eggs grits coffee	Bloated Sluggish Sleepy
1/1/00	1:15 PM	green salad tuna sandwich on whole grain bread fruit	Energized Satisfied Light
1/1/00	5:30 PM	rice steamed veggies fish	Satisfied
1/2/00	8:45 AM	oatmeal 1 slice toast 8 oz. orange juice	Satisfied
1/2/00	1 PM	hamburger french fries soda	Full Sluggish Tired
1/2/00	5 PM	green salad	Hungry

CHAPTER 11

Diet Confusion

African Americans are not the only people confused about diet. Today, everyone is bombarded 24/7 by television, radio, and print media with contradictory advertisements and reports about food, causing mass confusion about what to eat, what not to eat and why.

I am not surprised that we are in such a quandary because the recommendations about nutrition are forever changing. By the time we hear that a certain food or diet or supplement is good for us, someone else comes along and tells us that it is bad, and vice versa. Trying to decipher the information that we receive about food can be quite a dilemma.

The diet dilemma

It is no secret that the media has a direct influence on our poor eating habits, and feeds into our obsession about weight and beauty. So many commercials on television are about food, or, contrarily, offer the latest, best way to stay slim and trim. And it's important "news" when Janet Jackson, Oprah, or Al Roker gain or lose a few sizes.

Manufacturers of supplements are offering vitamins with "weight reduction properties," and even the beverage industry is getting in on the act with "low calorie" alcohol drinks.

There are an amazing number of weight-reducing products on the market. People have become so engrossed in this diet mania that conversations about food gravitate to carbs, calories, and weight status. The fact that the primary purpose of food is to nourish our bodies and keep us alive is usually not part of the discussion.

Advertisers try to convince you that their particular diet is better, or that a special "pill-a-day" will keep the pounds away. They imply *"you can eat anything you want"* and still drop weight.

A couple of years ago I was a guest speaker at a conference. During the conference break there were vendors selling items such as candles, books, and health products. In front of one vendor's booth was a big picture display of colorful fruits and vegetables.

So I strolled over to see what was being offered. The vendor was selling a bottle of capsules that claimed to provide all of the nutrients needed to maintain health, help you to lose weight, and cure diabetes, high blood pressure, and other ailments. Even more recently I attended a health seminar where someone approached me selling "whole" food nutrition fruits and vegetables in a *capsule*.

Because many people prefer the "quick fix" method to weight loss and nourishment, they are attracted to products that claim to provide everything in one capsule or dose. Some people will replace nourishing foods and even their medications with these products.

They feed on your food weaknesses because they are aware that most people, especially overweight people, love to eat; and will do almost anything as long as they don't have to give up their favorite junk foods. So, you are enticed with sugary desserts, and foods that are high in fats and sodium. And guess what? As a special treat they will throw in all of the diabetes, heart disease, and high blood pressure that you want on your plates, as well. In other words, you cannot get away with having your cake and eating it too. No pun intended.

Fad diets have been around for a long time—when one goes out another comes in. According to a recent 12-month study of four popular commercial diets, Atkins, Ornish, Zone and LEARN diets, the volunteers on the Atkins diet lost the most weight. But, all diets were similar in that after a few months the dieters began to pack on the pounds again regardless of the plan they followed.

The vegetarian dilemma

In the past being a vegetarian meant that you only consumed plant-based foods like fruits, vegetables, nuts and whole grains. This is not the case anymore. Today, there are so many categories of vegetarians that it is difficult to identify who is a vegetarian and who is not. Here are a few categories:

- **Vegan vegetarians**-eat only plant foods, no animal flesh, including fish, eggs, dairy products, or honey.
- **Lacto-vegetarians**-eat no animal flesh but include dairy products in their diets.
- **Ovo-vegetarians**-eat no animal flesh but include eggs in their diets.
- **Lacto-ovo vegetarians**-eat no animal flesh but include dairy products and eggs in their diets.
- **Pesco-vegetarians**-eat fish, eggs, and dairy products.
- **Pollo-vegetarians**-eat poultry, such as chicken, turkey, and duck.

Since the meaning of vegetarian has expanded far beyond that of plant-based foods, being a vegetarian does not necessarily mean that you are eating a healthy wholesome diet.

When some people become vegetarians they replace meat with refined foods like white rice, pasta, and processed vegetarian foods that look and taste like meat, but some of them contain the same harmful food additives as other processed foods. In addition, many who eat animal products and refined foods are overweight, have a high fat intake, high calorie intake, and have cholesterol problems just like non-vegetarians.

Actually, categorizing vegetarian diets was quite a brilliant ploy. I don't know who came up with the idea but it has certainly helped the meat and dairy industry stay prosperous. It is a clever way of encouraging people to eat animal products while giving them the false impression that they are vegetarians. Wow, what a concept!

The coffee dilemma

Is coffee good for you or is it bad for you? It depends on whom you ask. We hear reports that the caffeine in coffee is an addictive drug that causes tremendous headaches when you withdraw from consuming it. It also has been found to be bad for the cardiovascular system by making people more susceptible to heart disease, stroke, and increased cholesterol levels. In addition, pregnant women who drink coffee increase their chances of miscarriage by 36 percent. Coffee has also been found to contribute to anxiety, sleep disorders, high blood pressure, heartburn, and other physical problems.

On the other hand, some reports say that coffee is good for you, and that the key is to drink it in moderation. Coffee can increase your energy, enhance your mood, and may lesson the risks of certain diseases like Alzheimer's. Those who drink coffee are less likely to commit suicide, suffer from cirrhosis of the liver, develop diabetes, and coffee can lower the risk of gallstones by 40 percent.

An example of a contradictory "special report" about coffee is one that I saw on television. The report was about a study that says coffee may prevent men from getting diabetes. The report offered limited information, and did not explain how the men were selected for the study, or other factors that may have contributed to these men not getting diabetes, such as their lifestyle. At the end of the segment, the commentator issued a disclaimer stating that the results of the study were inconclusive.

Generally people do not pay attention to disclaimers, and they certainly are not privy to the full study. But because it was a "special report," some men may think that it is based on scientific conclusive evidence. As a result, they may consume larger amounts of coffee believing that it will protect them from diabetes.

Whether you drink coffee or not is a personal choice. You can drink it and increase your risk of developing anxiety, sleep disorder, or cardiovascular problems, or you can drink non-caffeinated beverages such as herbal teas and water and not have to worry about possible side effects of coffee.

The egg dilemma

Are eggs good or bad for you? This also depends on whom you ask. Some experts say that you should avoid eggs because they cause your cholesterol to elevate to dangerous levels, putting you at risk for coronary artery disease, and other cardiovascular risks.

On the other hand, there are experts declaring eggs are a perfect source of protein, vitamin A, Vitamin D, and riboflavin; and that they are good if eaten in moderation. Even the meaning of the term "moderation" changes—sometimes it means 1 or 2 eggs a week, and other times it means 3 or 4 eggs a week.

I say if you are not at risk for cardiovascular disease, you can probably get away with eating eggs in moderation. But if you are at risk for cardiovascular disease, you are probably better off eating the egg whites and not the yolk, which is mostly fat. And, try foods that provide some of the same protein and vitamins as eggs, such as green leafy vegetables and fish.

Don't believe the hype

For some people, if they see it on TV, *then it must be true*. When some people go grocery shopping, they seem to be choosing foods unconsciously as if they can hear familiar jingles from commercials buzzing in their ears, directing them to certain foods. Their attachment to food is basically emotional and induced by advertisement. They load their shopping carts with a variety of colorful prepackaged foods that are saturated with unhealthy artificial food additives used to enhance taste, add color, or maintain freshness. But because the foods taste so good, they don't consider what these foods are doing to their health.

When television begins to have that much influence on your eating habits, and becomes the primary source of information about how and what you eat, I suggest that you TURN OFF THE TV. At least stop watching the hypnotizing commercials. It is my opinion that most commercials about food do little more than encourage eating habits that lead to disease and illness.

Understand that the primary goal of food and beverage commercials is *to sell the product*—not to educate you about what's healthy. If this means that the advocates of these products give you mixed and/or false information to reach that goal, then that is what they will do—they don't have to pay your doctor bills.

It is important that you educate yourself about healthy eating so that you are acting in your own interest, and not the interest of others. You can do this by increasing your knowledge about nutrition, finding healthy diet alternatives, and listening to your own body.

This does not mean that you have to take classes or earn a degree in nutrition. But you should have basic knowledge about how to get the essential nutrients your body must have to stay vibrant and healthy. (See chapter 14 for antioxidant foods that are good for your body.)

CHAPTER 12

Reduce the Junk in Your Trunk

Being *"overweight"* refers to an excess of body weight that includes muscle, bone, fat, and water. Being *"obese"* refers specifically to having an abnormally high proportion of body fat. Today obesity is one of the critical health issues facing African Americans. It is estimated that about 75% of African Americans are now overweight or obese. This horrifying statistic is associated with many illnesses that plague our community.

The incidence of obesity among African Americans is partly due to socio-cultural differences in attitudes.

Many studies have shown that, in general, African Americans accept larger body sizes, and are more likely to refer to themselves as "a little heavy" or "big boned." A new study by Dana-Farber Cancer Institute reports that "overweight black Americans are two to three times more likely to say their weight is average—even after they've been diagnosed as overweight or obese by a doctor."

Black men are known to say that black women have more sex appeal when they have "meat on their bones," or "a little junk in the trunk." The more popular term today is "baby got back" or "cakes." This is all said in admiration of a black woman's pronounced behind.

It is no doubt that black men are more attracted to heavier women. As a matter of fact, even when they date outside their race, they tend to choose women with large body frames.

Overweight black men are proud of their own husky "teddy bear" look, and their "big guts." But the excess fat that they carry around their waistline can be dangerous. The shape of a person's body, as well as their body weight, can be indicators of their risk for cardiovascular disease. Some studies have shown that people with "apple shaped" bodies, or more fat distributed at the waistline, may have a higher risk of heart disease than people with "pear shaped" bodies, or more fat at the thigh or hips.

Who can't deny that a pear-shaped figure with an "itty-bitty" waistline and a noticeable backside is an admirable attribute to many men. Having a big behind is so vital to some black women that if they had to choose between losing weight at the expense of losing their behinds, they would opt for the bigger trunk. The problem is that when the fat in a black woman's butt expands, the fat in other parts of her body will expand as well. In the U.S. black women have the highest prevalence of being overweight and obese.

The standard of beauty and attractiveness that African Americans have set for themselves puts them at higher risk for chronic disease. Excess body weight increases the risks for premature death, hypertension, Type II diabetes, cardiovascular disease, stroke, gall bladder disease, respiratory problems, gout, osteoarthritis, some kinds of cancer, and premature death.

The most common way to find out whether you're overweight or obese is to figure out your body mass index (BMI). The BMI is a estimate of body fat and a good gauge of your risk for diseases that occur with more body fat. The higher your BMI, the higher the risk of disease. BMI is calculated from your height and weight. If your BMI is 25 - 29.9 you are overweight. If it is 30 or greater, you are obese. You can find out what your BMI is on the National Institute of Health BMI calculator at www.nhlbisupport.com/bmi.

High incidence of obesity, however, is not restricted to African American adults. Today there is a high rate of obesity among children. Overweight adolescents have a 70 percent chance of becoming overweight or obese adults. This increases to 80 percent if one or both parents are overweight or obese. The Department of Health and Human Services reports that the proportion of overweight children and adolescents ages 6-19 increased from 11 percent in 1988-1994 to 15 percent in 1999-2000. For black children and adolescents, the rates increased 22 percent.

The Institute of Medicine reports that the current increase of obesity is especially evident among ethnic minority populations—African American, Hispanic, and American Indians. Among boys, the highest prevalence of obesity is observed in Hispanic and among girls, the highest prevalence is observed in African Americans.

Causing more confusion for youth today is the hip-hop and R&B industry praising obesity. I recall seeing a popular television show featuring "fat and sexy" African American recording artists. As I watched the show I thought—*how many of these young black men will be alive or in good health by the time they reach their 60th birthday?* A lucky few. Gerald Lavert, my favorite young R&B singer, was one of the guest. (Tears came to my eyes when I heard that he had died recently at age 40 from a heart attack.)

Recent reports have also found that the current obesity rates of children could lower life expectancy, and lead to diseases that are normally seen in adults, such as diabetes, stroke, heart disease, and cancer.

Maintaining a healthy weight is a challenge in our society. And, decreasing the amount that you eat can be a difficult task given the trend of today's super-sized servings, such as 32-oz sodas, large orders of French fries, triple-layered burgers, table-size pizzas, and all-you-can-eat buffets.

But it is important to understand that losing even a small amount of weight can make big improvements in your health. For example, if you lose just ten pounds, and get thirty minutes of exercise a day, you can reduce your risk for diabetes and other serious illnesses.

If you put into practice the following healthy options for maintaining your ideal weight, you not only reduce your risk of disease, but look and feel better about yourself as well.

Healthy options for maintaining your ideal weight

Control your food portions

Be moderate in what you eat, even with good-for-you foods. Reduce your calorie intake by reducing the amount of food you put on your plate and put in your mouth. This is called "portion control." Studies have shown a relationship between increased portion sizes and obesity. Did you know that the portion size you are used to may be equal to two or three standard servings? For example, if a package of cookies lists one serving equals two cookies, and you eat four cookies, you are eating double the calories, fat, carbs, etc. (See example of serving sizes and portion sizes at the end of this section.)

Aim for a slow and steady weight loss

Slow, steady changes give you the best chance to reach and maintain a healthy weight. Decrease your portion size gradually so that your brain and your stomach will be less likely to notice the change. Even the smallest reduction on a continuing basis will add up to weight loss.

Exercise regularly

Physical activity is such an important part of weight management. The best way to lose weight is a combination of eating less and exercising. Studies have shown that people who lose weight and continue to exercise after reaching their target weight are more successful than people who do not exercise.

Eat meals and snacks low in fat

Fat has over twice the calories as carbohydrates or protein. If you eat low-fat foods, you can still eat well. But keep your calories under control. For example, snacking on fruits and vegetables that are low in calories and fat but high in fiber, keeps you feeling full longer, thus helping to prevent overeating. In addition, they are low in sodium, causing less water retention.

Eat out carefully

Restaurants generally serve very large portions. Instead of eating all of the food that is served, eat only half your meal and take the other half for lunch the next day. If you have dessert, split it with a friend. Ask for substitutions (steamed vegetables or salad instead of fries). And get your sauces, dressings, and gravies on the side so that you will be in control of the amount that is added to your plate. At buffets, be aware of how much food you pile on your plate and into your stomach.

Avoid fast foods

Fast foods may taste good and cost less but they are high in fat, sugar, and calories, and low in fiber. As such, they are known to cause excessive weight gain, contributing to obesity, diabetes, heart problems, and other conditions. If you must eat at a fast food chain, choose foods that are not fried, salads, and low fat dressings on the side.

Don't crash diet

A crash diet is a very low calorie diet designed to make you lose weight in a short amount of time. Crash diets actually starve your body of nutrients. This causes the cells in your body to become sluggish, and slows down your metabolism, *actually encouraging weight gain.* The large majority of people who go on crash diets gain back every ounce of the weight they have lost, and more.

Monitor your eating behavior

Keep these questions in mind each time you reach for something to eat: *Do you eat for pleasure or are you a food connoisseur? Are you satisfying a craving? Are you just bored? Do you eat to fulfill an emotional need? Do you eat when you are not hungry or overindulge in foods without real-izing it?* It is important to take note of *hidden motivators* that contribute to overeating and weight gain.

Keep a food diary

Writing down everything you eat will make you more aware of eating habits and patterns that you may not have noticed, or try to ignore. Studies have shown that keeping track of what you eat can help you make changes in your diet, and is vital to successful weight control. Be sure to note exactly when, what, and how much you eat. (See a sample Food Diary at the end of this section).

Get support

Adjusting to a new way of eating will be easier if you get the support of others. Team up with a family member or friend who can share your interest in healthy eating. Seek out groups and organizations that can provide information and guidance about healthy eating. Hit the Internet, library and bookstores for fitness guides and healthy menu planning.

Set realistic goals

Don't expect the impossible! There is no magic for losing weight. The optimal way to lose weight and keep it off is through *permanent lifestyle changes.*

PORTION SIZE EXAMPLES

- 3-4 ounces of meat is the size of a deck of cards or a medium bar of soap

- 1 ounce of meat is the size of a matchbox

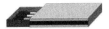

- 3 ounces of fish is the size of a checkbook

- 1 ounce of cheese is the size of four dice

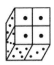

- A medium potato is the size of a computer mouse

- 2 Tbs. of peanut butter is the size of a ping-pong ball

- 1 cup of pasta is the size of a tennis ball

Source: American Cancer Society

WHAT COUNTS AS A SERVING?
Examples of one serving size

Milk Group
1 cup (8 oz) milk or yogurt
2 slices cheese, 1/8" thick (1½ oz)
1½ cups ice milk, ice cream, or frozen yogurt

Meat & Meat Alternatives Group
2-3 oz cooked lean meat, poultry, or fish
2 eggs
7 oz tofu
1 cup cooked legumes (dried beans or peas)
½ cup nuts or seeds

Vegetable Group
½ cup cooked vegetables
½ cup raw vegetables
1 cup raw leafy vegetables
½ to ¾ cup vegetable juice

Fruit Group
1 whole medium fruit (about 1 cup)
¼ cup dried fruit
½ cup canned fruit
½ to ¾ cup fruit juice

Grain Group
1 slice bread
½ bagel or English muffin
4 small crackers
1 tortilla
½ cup cooked cereal
½ hot dog bun or hamburger bun
1 teaspoon oil, margarine, or butter

1 medium muffin
½ cup pasta
1 cup cold cereal
½ cup rice

Sample

FOOD DIARY

DAY OF WEEK: _____

TIME	FOOD - BEVERAGE	HOW MUCH	WHERE
7:15 AM	coffee with sugar toast with raspberry jam	2 cups 3 pieces	At home
10:20 AM	Red Bull trail mix	can 8 oz	In the car after stopping at 7-11
12:20 PM	hamburger French fries Coke	1 double cheese 1 large 1 16 oz.	McDonalds
3:45 PM	Snickers bottled water green grapes	2 reg. size 1 large 2 handfuls	Front of the computer at home
6:50 PM	pizza-the works beer pecan ice cream	4 slices 2 bottles Bud 3 scoops & syrup	At a friend's house
10:45 PM	chips and dip Seven-up	½ bag bar-b-q 1 can	Watching TV at home

CHAPTER 13

Variety is the Spice of Life

Many of us get in the habit of eating the same foods over and over without venturing to try something new. When we stick to favorites and limit variety, we also limit the ability to get a balance of nutrients.

No one food group contains all of the essential nutrients, and a growing list of disease-fighting antioxidants (discussed later) are needed to ensure that you have optimum health and vitality. This is why it is necessary to eat a variety of foods to ensure that you are getting everything your body needs.

An example of how foods are different in their nutrient value is the content of an orange compared to cheese. The orange provides vitamin C and folate but no vitamin B, or cheese, which provides calcium and vitamin B but no vitamin C.

There are six essential nutrients that you must have in order to live:

- Proteins
- Carbohydrates
- Fats
- Vitamins
- Minerals
- Water

Without a variety from these six nutrient groups your body does not receive the proper fuel it needs to function optimally and you *will* develop health problems.

Each nutrient has at least one specific job, and unfortunately nutrients can't cover for each other. When your body is deprived of any one of these essential nutrients, your immune system is weakened, leaving you vulnerable to illness and disease.

- **Protein:** Protein is the building blocks of your body. Dietary protein provides the amino acids (protein units) that help build muscle, skin, blood, hair, nails, and internal organs.
- **Carbohydrates:** Starches and sugars are the major carbohydrates. Carbohydrates are the body's key source of energy and are critical in helping to maintain tissue protein and to metabolize fat. All carbo-

hydrates are ultimately broken down into glucose (blood sugar) to fuel the cells of your body.

- **Fats:** Fat is a major source of energy for your body and is necessary for the absorption of vitamins A, D, E, and K. Certain fatty acids are necessary for life, growth, and healthy organs and skin. Your body uses fat to manufacture sex hormones, skin oil, bile, cushions vital organs and nerves, and protects you from extreme cold and heat.

- **Vitamins:** They have many functions including enhancing your body's use of carbohydrates, proteins, and fats. They are critical in the formation of blood cells, hormones, and nervous system chemicals.

- **Minerals:** They are very small amounts of metallic elements that are vital for the healthy growth of teeth and bones. They are the building blocks for other cells and enzymes. Minerals help to regulate the balance of fluids in your body, and control the movement of nerve impulses.

- **Water:** Water is classified as a vital nutrient just like protein, carbohydrates, fats, vitamins and minerals. In order to live, every cell in your body must be bathed in water. Water is a major component of your blood, which transports all the other nutrients in your cells, and toxins and waste out of your body. (See chapter 20, Turn on the Water Works.)

Dietary guidelines for healthy eating

An easy way to get a variety of foods to ensure you get a balance of the essential nutrients discussed above, is to select foods and beverages within the five basic food groups as outlined in the 2005 Dietary Guidelines for America.

The food groups are:

- Grain group
- Vegetable group
- Fruit group
- Milk group
- Meat & Bean group

The basic premise of these guidelines is that nutrient needs should be met primarily through consuming foods.

The recommendations suggested in each food group are for people (adults) eating 2,000 calories a day, with higher or lower amounts depending on calorie intake.

- *Foods in the grain group:* Any food made from wheat, rice, oats, cornmeal, barley or another cereal grain is a grain product. Bread, pasta, oatmeal, tortillas, and hominy grits, corn bread, biscuits, rice, and hush puppies, are examples of grain products. *Recommendation is to eat 6 oz. of grains every day. Half of your grains (3 oz.) should be whole grains.*
- *Foods in the vegetable group:* Any vegetable or 100 percent vegetable juice counts as a member of the vegetable group. Vegetables may be raw or cooked; fresh, frozen, canned, or dried/dehydrated; and may be whole, cut-up or mashed. Greens, turnips, succotash, corn, sweet potatoes, okra, cabbage, are examples of vegetable products. *Recommendation is to eat 2 ½ cups every day.*

- *Foods in the fruit group:* Any fruit or 100 percent fruit juice counts as part of the fruit group. Fruits may be fresh, canned, frozen, or dried, and may be whole, cut-up, or pureed. *Recommendation is to eat 2 cups every day.*

- *Foods in the milk group:* Any fluid milk products and many foods made from milk are considered part of this food group. Foods made from milk that retain their calcium content are part of this group, while foods made from milk that have little to no calcium, such as cream cheese, cream, and butter, are not.

  Many African Americans do not have the lactase enzyme to digest milk or milk products. This is called "lactose intolerance." If you have trouble digesting dairy products, you can buy lactose-free milk, milk with lactase enzymes added to it, or you can use soymilk and soy products. Soymilk and soy products are also alternatives for people like vegetarians who do not eat animal products. *Recommendation is to consume 3 cups every day.*

- *Foods in the meat & beans group:* Any foods made from meat, poultry, fish, dry beans or peas, eggs, nuts, and seeds are considered part of this protein group. Dry beans and peas are part of this group as well as the vegetable group.

Plant proteins found in vegetables, grains and legumes (beans and peas) are not complete proteins and cannot support growth by themselves. However, when served in the proper combination, plant proteins can provide all of the essential amino acids without the addition of animal protein. A good example is beans and rice. Each of these foods lack one or more essential amino acids, but the amino acids missing in rice are found in beans, and vice versa. When eaten together, these foods provide a complete source of protein.

Other examples are: Brown rice combined with peas; Whole wheat pasta combined with broccoli; Whole wheat bread combined with potato stew; Whole wheat bread combined with peanut butter (sandwich).

Recommendation for eating foods in the meat & beans group is 5½ oz. every day.

As you increase your knowledge and understanding of what food nutrients are and why they are important, I believe you will be much better motivated to make healthier food choices.

CHAPTER 14

Complexity is Good for the Body

Does your plate typically display a sizable portion of meat, one (small serving) of vegetable, and a starch such as potatoes or rice? Or maybe you pile your plate with two kinds of meat, like spaghetti with ground meat, and fried chicken?

Like many Americans, African American meals are *meat centered,* and often extremely low in fruits, vegetables, and whole grain products. Few people realize that vegetables and grains are not considered side dishes, but are essential to a balanced meal.

To balance your plate, incorporate a variety of *complex* carbohydrates (vegetables, fruits, and whole grains) and less animal foods (meats, eggs, and dairy products). As a matter of fact, the American Institute of Cancer Research (AICR) recommends a plate with two-thirds or more vegetables, fruits, whole grains and beans, and one-third or less of animal protein.

Two types of carbohydrates

There are two types of carbs: *Complex carbohydrates* (starches), and *simple carbohydrates* (sugars). However, regardless of the type of carbohydrate, your body will convert all carbohydrates, starches and sugars, to sugar glucose. (Glucose is a type of sugar that comes from digesting carbohydrates into a chemical that we can easily convert to energy). Each gram of carbohydrates, by the way, generates four calories.

Complex carbohydrates (or complex sugars) are made up of hundreds or thousands of sugar units. Main sources of complex carbohydrates are foods such as potatoes, vegetables, beans, peas, and brown rice. Complex carbohydrates are digested and absorbed by your body slowly. This slow absorption results in a steady blood sugar level, which allows you to feel full longer and gives you lasting energy, while regulating your blood sugar and insulin levels.

Simple carbohydrates (or simple sugars), on the other hand, are made up of one or two sugar units. Simple carbohydrates are mainly added sugars, which have very little nutritional value. Examples of simple carbohydrates are soda, white bread, and candy, etc. Fruit is also considered a simple carbohydrate, but fruit has the benefit of being rich in vitamins, minerals and fiber.

Simple carbohydrates are digested and absorbed by your body rapidly, setting off a chain of unhealthy events discussed in chapter 17.

Eating plenty of fruits and vegetables and grains (grains are discussed in more detail in chapter 15) can help reduce your risk of developing heart disease, certain cancers, and other chronic diseases. They contain all of the vitamins, minerals, and enzymes that you need to help maintain your health and are also low in fat and sodium. For example, a slice of whole wheat bread will provide you with B vitamins, zinc, and some protein. In addition, they are packed with **fiber**.

Fiber has been linked to a reduced risk of colon cancer; it lowers your cholesterol, and is essential for healthy digestive functions.

As the saying goes, "There is a reason for everything," and there are healthy reasons to eat a rainbow of colorful fruits and vegetables. Each color fruit and vegetable offers different vitamins and minerals. (See vitamin and mineral charts in chapter 19)

And, each fruit and vegetable is rich in **antioxidants**, which are plant substances that can help prevent diseases like heart disease and cancer, and slow the effects of aging. These naturally-occurring substances protect the body from harmful excess "free radicals" (unstable oxygen molecules) by sweeping them up before they can cause damage to your cells. The best way to have a rich antioxidant foundation that protects you from toxins and free radicals is through a combination of **whole foods.**

Whole foods (unprocessed foods in their natural state), fruits, vegetables, and grains—not pills or supplements—can give you these health benefits. In other words, God has figured it all out for us; all we have to do is eat and enjoy!

God's rainbow of food colors

Orange/yellow fruits and vegetables contain powerful antioxidants such as vitamin C, carotenoids, and bioflavonoids, which provide the following health benefits:

- Reduces the risk of heart disease
- Reduces the risk of certain cancers
- Improves the immune system
- Helps maintain healthy eyes

Examples of orange/yellow fruits and vegetables:

carrots	pumpkins	peaches
oranges	lemons	squash
apricots	cantaloupes	mangoes
corn	pineapple	sweet potatoes
nectarines	rutabagas	tangerines
grapefruit	persimmons	apricots

Red fruits and vegetables contain the antioxidants lycopene and anthrocyanins, which provide the following health benefits:

- Protects against ultraviolet rays
- Reduces the risk of certain cancers
- Improves memory function

- Helps maintain urinary tract health
- Helps maintain heart health

Examples of red fruits and vegetables:

red apples	beets	red cabbage
cherries	cranberries	red grapes
radishes	watermelon	strawberries
tomatoes	red peppers	red potatoes
raspberries	pomegranates	pink grapefruit
rhubarb		

Green fruits and vegetables contain the antioxidants luthein and zeaxanthin, which provide the following health benefits:

- Reduces your risk of cataracts and age-related macular degeneration, which can lead to blindness
- Reduces the risk of certain cancers
- Helps maintain strong bones and teeth

Examples of green fruits and vegetables:

green apples	artichokes	asparagus
avocadoes	green beans	broccoli
Brussels sprouts	cabbage	green grapes
lettuce	cucumbers	limes
honeydew melon	kiwi	green pepper
green onions	peas	collard greens
spinach	zucchini	

Blue/purple fruits and vegetables contain the antioxidants anthocyanins and phenolics, which provide the following health benefits:

- Improves memory
- Reduces the of risk of some cancers
- Promotes healthy aging
- Help maintain urinary tract health

Examples of blue/purple fruits and vegetables:

blackberries	blueberries	eggplant
figs	purple cabbage	plums
prunes	purple grapes	raisins

White fruits and vegetables contain the antioxidant Allicin, which provides the following health benefits:

- Helps lower cholesterol
- Helps lower blood pressure
- Reduces the risk of some cancers
- Reduces the risk of heart disease

Examples of white fruits and vegetables:

bananas	cauliflower	garlic
ginger	jicama	mushrooms
onions	parsnips	white potatoes
turnips	white nectarines	white peaches
white corn		

Healthy ways to prepare fruits and vegetables

- Eat vegetables raw, steamed, frozen, and as lightly-cooked as possible. High temperatures causes loss of nutrients and enzymes. Use the nutritious liquid "pot likker" left from cooking for soups, stews, and sauces.
- Use herbs and spices for flavoring vegetables instead of fatty meats. (See list of herbs and spices described in chapter 18).
- Avoid frying vegetables in large amounts of butter or oil. (Stir frying uses little oil).
- Switch from iceberg lettuce, which lacks nutrients and taste, to romaine or other dark leaf lettuces that have more fiber, vitamins, and minerals.
- Eat fruits and vegetables for snacks.
- Serve fruits for desserts and to make smoothies.
- Eat fruits and vegetables in season whenever possible. Fruits and vegetables are most nutritious and taste best when they are picked at their peak.
- Buy organically grown produce whenever possible. Organic food is grown, processed, and packaged without the use of agricultural chemicals, artificial colors, or flavors, genetic modification, irradiation, or other synthetic ingredients.
- Eat 2-4 servings of fruits a day.
- Eat 3-5 servings of vegetables a day.

Healthy Vegetable and Fruit Recipes

Down-Home Meatless Greens
(Inspired by Mary Barnes)

3 bunches collard greens
1 bunch kale greens
1 bunch chard greens
1½ cups Italian dressing
2 cup water
1 Tbsp. apple cider vinegar
1 Tbsp. olive oil
1 tsp. sea salt (optional)

1. Wash the greens and cut out the rib. Cut the greens into small pieces and set aside.
2. In a large pot, mix the remaining ingredients and let simmer over medium heat for 2-3 minutes.
3. Add the greens to the mixture and bring to a boil. Turn the heat to low and cook until tender. Stir occasionally adding small amounts of water if necessary.

Note: You can use your own favorite Italian dressing. My favorite is "Cardini" Italian or lemon herb. Be careful when adding salt because most salad dressings have quite a bit of sodium in them already.

Tasty Steamed Mixed Vegetables

2 medium carrots
6 broccoli florets
1 medium zucchini squash
1 cup Italian dressing
½ tsp. basil
½ tsp. oregano

1. Cut carrots and zucchini into small pieces.
2. In a large plastic zip-lock baggie, mix the Italian dressing and seasoning.
3. Place the vegetables in the baggie and shake well. Let them marinate in the mixture for 20 minutes. Remove the vegetables from the baggie and place in a vegetable steamer. Steam until slightly tender.

Vegetable Juice Drink

3 medium carrots
1 celery stalk
1 cucumber

1. Wash and cut the vegetables into medium pieces.
2. Place ingredients in the juicer.
3. Serve chilled.

Mixed Fruit Smoothie

1 medium banana
1 medium peach
½ cup blueberries
1 cup soymilk

1. Peel banana and cut into small pieces.
2. Cut peach into small pieces. Discard the seed.
3. Place all ingredients in a blender. Blend until smooth. Add more milk if you want less thickness.

Note: Any combination of fresh or frozen fruit can be used for variety. Including bananas gives the smoothie a thicker smooth consistency and adds sweetness.

Note: A great place to find reasonably-priced produce in season is at the USDA Farmers Markets. You can have access to locally grown, farm-fresh produce and the opportunity to personally interact with the farmer who grows the produce. To find a listing of farmers markets in your state or local area:

- call 1-800-384-8704 or
- visit the website:
www.ams.usda.gov/farmersmarket/map.htm

CHAPTER 15

All Grains are Not the Same

Whole grains are complex carbohydrates. Like fruits and vegetables, they are rich in disease-fighting antioxidants, and loaded with vital nutrients such as protein, magnesium, thiamin, riboflavin, niacin, iron, vitamin A, B, C, protein, and fiber. Although whole grains cannot be identified by the color of the food, they come in many shapes and sizes, from large kernels of popcorn to small quinoa seeds.

Because they are so rich in fiber, whole grains are mostly associated with providing roughage in the diet, preventing constipation, hemorrhoids, and diverticulosis disease (small pouches in the colon caused by low fiber diet); and keeping the overall digestive system healthy.

- 100g of cooked long-grain white rice = 0.5g of fiber.
- 100g of cooked long-grain brown rice = 1.5g of fiber

Eating whole grains, as well as foods made from them, has also been shown to have many other great health benefits, such as reducing the risk of heart disease, stroke, cancer, diabetes, and obesity.

Whole grains, as in whole wheat flour, consist of the entire grain seed called the kernel. The kernel contains germ and bran that are rich in dietary fiber, vitamins, minerals, and other vital nutrients. Refining whole wheat into white flour removes the nutritious germ and bran, and is no longer whole wheat.

Refinement is intended to increase shelf life and lighten the product. Just because a slice of bread is dark does not guarantee that it was made from whole wheat. Some bread labeled "wheat" is actually white bread with molasses added to give it a darker color. So please be aware that if a product does not say "*whole* wheat" or "*whole* grain" as the first ingredient listed on the food label, it is a refined product that has been stripped of most of the nutrient value.

When you see the word "enriched" on foods made from grains, it means that vitamins and minerals that were removed during the refining process have been added back into it. However, enrichment only restores a *portion* of what was lost during the processing of the original whole grain.

Many African Americans eat less than one daily serving of whole grains, and many never eat whole grain foods at all. Eating the daily recommended amount of grains each day (6 oz.) is actually not as hard as it seems. One serving of whole grains is equal to:

½ cup cooked or 1 ounce of ready-to-eat cereal
1 slice whole grain bread
5 to 7 small whole grain crackers
½ cup whole grain pasta or brown rice
2 cups of popcorn

Here are examples of whole grain foods, plus healthy ways to incorporate them into your diet.

Types of whole grain foods

barley	millet
buckwheat	oatmeal
brown rice	popcorn
whole wheat bread	quinoa
whole wheat pasta	whole wheat crackers
flaxseed	

Healthy options for eating whole grains

- Substitute whole wheat toast for bagels.
- Substitute low-fat, multigrain muffins for pastries.
- Eat brown rice instead of white rice. Brown rice is also chewier and has more flavor.
- Substitute half of all-purpose flour with whole wheat when baking breads or cookies.

- Eat whole wheat or whole grain bread instead of white bread.
- Eat whole grain or whole wheat cereals instead of sugar-coated cereals. Try bran flakes, shredded wheat or oatmeal.
- Enjoy low fat whole grain crackers, baked tortilla chips or brown rice cake as a snack.
- Eat whole grain pasta (macaroni, spaghetti, noodles), pancakes or waffles for a change of pace.
- Serve grains with beans for a complete protein meal, as a side dish, in casseroles, stews, or soups, or as a hot cereal.
- **Quinoa** is a good substitute for rice, and quinoa flour is a replacement for white flour in baked goods. It can also be cooked and used in salads, soups, and stews.
- **Barley** can be eaten in soups, stews, hot cereals and casseroles. Also try using barley in salads or stuffing.
- **Millet** can be used in salads, pilafs or mixed with pasta.
- **Flaxseed** (ground) can be sprinkled over salads, soups, yogurt, or cereal. It gives a wonderful nutty flavor. It is not technically a whole grain, but it has a simular vitamin and mineral profile to grains.

Experiment with new whole grain products. Replacing your unhealthy refined grains, such the white flour, white bread, and white pasta, with healthy whole grains, will give you excellent nutritional benefits as well as more variety in your diet.

CHAPTER 16

Fat is Greasy

During slavery white people lived what is called "high on the hog." From the proceeds of slavery, they reveled in the finest life had to offer, including what was considered during those times as the finest foods. While slaves were living "low on the hog," forced to consume the feet, intestines, and tail of the hog, whites sank their teeth into pork chops, lean bacon, and ham. Now that we too can live high on the hog, we are paying a much higher price with our health.

The typical African American diet contains an abundance of fat and grease. Foods such as deep-fried chicken, catfish, pork chops, and hot water cornbread are more popular than boiled or baked foods.

Although fats and oils are part of a healthy diet, the type and the amount of fat that you consume makes a difference for heart health. Eating excess fat increases your risk of dying prematurely from heart disease, and is also linked to diabetes, obesity, and cancers of the colon, prostate, breast, and uterus.

It is important to know about the fats you consume. Even though all types of fat contain the same amount of calories (one gram of all fats = 9 calories), they are not all created equal. Small amounts of some fats called "good fats" can be beneficial, while small amounts of other fats called "bad fats" can be detrimental. For example, some fats (discussed later) in your diet can have a negative effect on your blood cholesterol levels.

Cholesterol is a white waxy substance found in all the healthy cell membranes in your body. Cholesterol is vital to good health as it is important for the formation of brain and nervous tissue, vitamin D and a variety of hormones. Your liver produces most of the cholesterol in your body and supplies all of the cholesterol that you need.

Two main types of cholesterol

High-density lipoproteins (HDL) are referred to as "good" cholesterol because they take cholesterol out of your blood and keep it from building up in your artery walls. The higher level of HDL actually protects you against heart disease.

Low-density lipoproteins (LDL) are referred to as "bad" cholesterol because they deposit cholesterol in the wall of your arteries, which builds up, increasing your risk of getting heart disease.

When you combine the cholesterol that you consume from too much fat in your diet (called dietary cholesterol), with the cholesterol being produced by your body, your levels of cholesterol can get too high. Knowing which fats raise your blood cholesterol levels and which ones don't, and then making better choices, is a major step toward lowering your risk of heart disease.

According to The American Heart Association, there are three levels of total cholesterol that relate to the amount of risk you have for developing heart disease:

- *A desirable level of total cholesterol is less than 200 mg/dL*, meaning your risk for heart disease is average.
- A borderline high-risk for heart disease is when your total cholesterol level is 200-239 mg/dL.
- A high-risk level for heart disease occurs when the total your cholesterol level is 240 mg/dL or greater.

Food Sources of Dietary Cholesterol

Dairy products (cream, butter, ice cream, milk), egg yolks, fatty meats, and organ meats (liver, kidney, and brains).

Triglycerides

- Triglycerides are a type of fat found in your blood. They are a major source of energy and the most common type of fat in your body. Like cholesterol, they are essential for good health when in normal amounts. All extra calories (regardless of what kind) are turned into triglycerides and stored in your fat cells to be used later. High triglycerides are linked to an increased risk of heart disease, diabetes, and stroke.

The good fats

- *Mono-unsaturated fats* come from plant sources. They are usually liquid at room temperature but may start to solidify in the refrigerator. These fats have the best effect on blood cholesterol, decreasing the level of bad cholesterol and increasing the level of good cholesterol. Mono-unsaturated fats have been proven to be the safest source of fat because they reduce the risk of heart disease.

Food Sources of Mono-unsaturated Fats

Olive oil, canola oil, peanut oils. Avocados and most nuts also have high amounts of mono-unsaturated fats.

- *Poly-unsaturated fats* come from plant sources. They are usually liquid at room temperature and in the refrigerator. Polyunsaturated fats lower your bad cholesterol, and raise your good cholesterol. However, if consumed in excess it can also *decrease* your good cholesterol.

Food Sources of Polyunsaturated Fats

Sunflower and sesame seeds, soybean, corn, safflower oils, and cottonseed oils.

- *Omega-3 fatty acids* are a special type of poly-unsaturated fat. They are called essential fatty acids (EFA) because they are crucial for good health. However, since the body cannot make them on its own, omega-3s must be obtained from food. Omega-3s have been shown to play a major role in keeping cholesterol levels low, stabilizing irregular heartbeat, reducing blood pressure, and preventing coronary heart disease.

Food Sources of Omega-3 Fatty Acids

Cold-water fish such as salmon, sardines, tuna, mackerel, herring. Canola oil, flaxseed, flaxseed oil, walnuts, and green leafy vegetables.

The bad fats

- *Saturated fats* are usually solid at room temperature. Saturated fats are bad for you because they raise bad blood cholesterol the most. Over time, this extra cholesterol can clog your arteries, causing "hardening of the arteries." Your arteries become narrowed and blood flow to the heart is slowed down or blocked, putting you at risk for a major heart attack or stroke. Saturated fats are found primarily in foods that come from animal sources, but are also found in some plant foods.

Food Sources of Saturated Fat

Beef, veal, lamb, pork, lard, poultry fat, butter, cream, milk, cheeses and other dairy products made from whole milk, palm oil, palm kernel, coconut oil, and cocoa butter.

- *Trans fat* (trans-fatty acids) is made when food manufacturers add hydrogen to vegetable oil. This process, which is called hydrogenation, causes oil to become solid at room temperature. It also increases the shelf life of perishable foods, and adds flavor. Trans fats are a common ingredient in commercial baked goods such as piecrust (makes it flaky), crackers (keeps them crispy), pastries, snack foods, stick margarine, and fried foods. Meats, milk, and other animal products contain trans fats naturally.

  Trans fats are considered more harmful than saturated fat because they not only raise your bad cholesterol level, but also lower your good cholesterol level. Studies have linked trans fat to heart disease and high blood cholesterol. On food labels, look for the words "partially hydrogenated" in the list of ingredients to see if the product contains trans fat.

Food Sources of Trans Fat

Crackers, cookies, cakes, piecrust, doughnuts, French fries, and other fast (junk) foods, shortenings and stick margarines (not liquid).

When you consume a diet that is low in saturated fats, trans fat, and cholesterol, it will have a favorable effect on your total blood cholesterol levels.

It is recommended that you keep your total fat intake between 20 to 35 percent of calories. Of that, 10 percent or less should come from saturated fats; most fats coming from sources of polyunsaturated and monounsaturated fatty acids.

Cholesterol intake should be kept to less than 300 milligrams of cholesterol a day (the yolk of one large egg provides about 214 milligrams of cholesterol).

Keep trans fatty acid consumption as low as possible. Some nutritionists and other diet specialists believe that no level of trans fat consumption is safe.

There is currently no dietary recommendation for trans fatty acids. However, as of January 2005, it is mandatory that all manufacturers indicate on the food label if their products contain trans fat. Be aware that products with 0.5 grams of trans fat per serving are allowed to be labeled as zero ("0") grams of trans fat. This means that if you eat large portions, the amount of trans fat you consume can add up quickly. (See Interpreting Food Label Terms at the end of this section).

It's not necessary that you try to completely eliminate all fats from your diet because it is not possible. Rather, be sure to choose the best types of fat and eat it in moderation.

Healthy options for reducing fats

Meats, Poultry, and Fish

Instead of:

- Fatback and bacon
- Chitlins
- Hog maws
- Pig feet
- Beef oxtails
- Large portions of meat

Try this:

- Lean meats with visible fat trimmed
- Poultry without the skin
- Choose chicken breasts or drumsticks instead of wings and thighs
- Eat fish more often
- Eat beans and grain dishes for protein more often
- Eat less red meat. (Heavy consumption of red meat has been linked to colon and prostate cancer.)

Dairy Products

Instead of:

- Whole milk or whole milk products
- Regular mayonnaise
- Regular salad dressing

Try this:

- Skim (nonfat) or 1% milk
- Low-fat or part skim cheeses
- Evaporated skim milk
- Low-fat yogurt
- Fortified soymilk: Soymilk contains no cholesterol or hormones
- Add slices of avocado, rather than cheese, to your sandwiches

Fats, Spreads, and Dressings

Instead of:

- Lard
- Butter
- Shortening
- Hard stick margarine
- Regular mayonnaise
- Regular salad dressing

Try this:

- Vegetable oil in small amounts
- Mustard alone, or nonfat or low-fat salad dressing, yogurt, or mayonnaise

- Soft margarines (liquids or tub varieties), with no more than 2 grams of saturated fat per tablespoon, and non-hydrogenated trans fat free
- Snack on a handful of nuts and or seeds instead potato chips or processed crackers

Healthy-fat cooking tips

- Sauté with olive oil instead of butter.
- Use olive oil in salad dressings and marinades.
- Broil, boil, steam, and roast instead of deep fat fried or batter-dipped fried foods.
- For crispy fish: dip in low-fat Italian dressing, roll in cornmeal, and then bake.
- For crispy chicken: remove skin, dip in skim milk/herbs and spices mix, roll in cornflakes and bake.
- For cakes, cookies, quick breads, and pancakes: Use egg whites or egg substitute instead of whole eggs. Two egg whites can be substituted in many recipes for one whole egg.
- Use spices to season foods like beans and greens instead of high-fat pork products.
- Read the nutrition fact label to see how much fat and saturated fats are in each serving.

INTERPRETATION OF FOOD LABEL TERMS
Source: Food and Drug Administration (FDA)

ITEM	SPECIFICATIONS
LOW FAT	3 grams or less of fat per serving
LESS FAT	25% or less fats than comparison foods
FAT FREE	Less than 0.5 grams of fat per serving with no added fat or oil
SATURATED FAT FREE	Less than 0.5 grams of saturated fat, and 0.5 grams of trans-fatty acids per serving
CHOLESTEROL FREE	Less than 2 mg per serving, and 2 grams or less saturated fat per serving
LOW CALORIE	40 calories or less per serving
LOW CHOLESTEROL	20 mg or less cholesterol per serving, and 2 grams or less saturated fat per serving
REDUCED CALORIE	At least 25% fewer calories per serving than the comparison food
LEAN	Less than 10 grams of fat, 4.5 grams of saturated fat, and 95 mg of cholesterol per (100 gram) serving
EXTRA LEAN	Less than 5 grams of fat, 2 grams of saturated fat, and 95 mg of cholesterol per (100 gram) serving
LIGHT (FAT)	50% or less of fat than the comparison food
LIGHT (CALORIES)	1/3 fewer calories than the comparison food

ITEM	SPECIFICATIONS
Sugar-free	Less than 0.5 grams of sugar per serving
Low sodium	140 mg or less per serving
Very low sodium	35 mg or less per serving
Sodium free	Less than 5 mg of sodium per serving
High, rich in, or excellent source	20% or more of the (RDA) Recommended Daily Value per serving
High fiber	5 grams or more fiber per serving
Less, fewer or reduced	At least 25% less than the comparison food
Low or low source	Means an amount that allows frequent consumption without exceeding the Recommended Daily Value for the nutrient
Good source	Provides 10% of the Recommended Daily Value for a given nutrient than the comparison food
Healthy	Low in fat, saturated fat, cholesterol, and sodium. Contains at least 10% of the Recommended Daily Values for vitamin A, vitamin C, iron, calcium, protein, and/or fiber.
Fresh	(1) A food is raw, has never been frozen or heated, and contains no preservatives (irradiation at low levels is allowed) (2) The term accurately describes the product (e.g. "fresh milk" or "freshly baked bread")
Fresh frozen	The food has been quickly frozen while still fresh; blanching is allowed before freezing to prevent nutrient breakdown.

CHAPTER 17

Sugar and Spice Ain't Always Nice

Who could resist a down-home sock-it-to-me cake, or a lip-smacking peach cobbler layered with crispy crust, or a moist three-layer German chocolate cake? Not many of us.

Tasty sweets like these are frequently eaten in African American homes, especially during times of celebration. And, it is not uncommon for us to include a flavored drink with our favorite desserts (i.e., fruit juice, lemonade, Kool-Aid or soda loaded with sugar).

Sugars are *simple carbohydrates*. Simple carbohydrates include table sugar (sucrose), honey, fructose (sugar from fruit), and lactose (sugar from milk). Foods such as candy, jelly, syrup, cookies, soda, and pastries are made from refined simple carbohydrates.

Simple carbohydrates, unlike complex carbohydrates, require little digestion and are quickly absorbed by your body, which triggers a chain of unhealthy events in your body.

First, the rapid absorption of simple sugar causes a spike in your blood sugar level. This means that if your blood sugar was 80 or 90 before you drank the can of soda or devoured a candy bar, it can suddenly spike to 150, 200, or higher.

The rise in your blood sugar then sends a message to your body to secrete more insulin in order to handle the sugar overload. In turn, the surge of insulin that is poured into the bloodstream causes the blood sugar to drop too low; this results in feeling jittery, irritable, fatigued, hungry, and craving even more sugar shortly after you have eaten.

Having a high blood sugar level is very serious, especially for people with diabetes. If it is allowed to continue it will cause a condition known as "diabetic neuropathy," which means the nerves that feed various limbs in your body (feet mostly) start to *die*.

Many African Americans with Type II diabetes have had to have their feet or legs amputated because the nerves in their feet are wasted away.

According to the American Diabetes Association (ADA), many African Americans who have diabetes know they have it, but continue to eat their same diet. The onset of Type II diabetes among African Americans is 70 percent higher than for white Americans. A diet high in calories, being overweight or obese, and having an inactive lifestyle are the main risk factors for Type II diabetes.

The truth of the matter is that all Americans eat an excessive amount of sugar (mainly sucrose). The average American consumes nearly 150 pounds of sugar a year. The dietary intake of pastry has increased 70 percent since 1945, snack food 85 percent, and soft drinks 200 percent. This increased consumption of sugar in our diets has been implicated in the development of numerous diseases.

Refined sugars are high in calories and void of nutrients (vitamins, etc.) This is referred to as "empty calories" because refined foods are loaded with calories from sugar and fats but lack the essential nutrients that your body needs to maintain health (with the exception of fructose, which contains mostly simple sugars but offers vitamins, minerals and fiber).

Sugar is everywhere

Refined sugar is the most prevalent single food additive in the American diet. And it is very addictive, so, the more you eat, the more you want. Seventy-five percent of the sugar consumed in America is from processed and packaged foods and from restaurants and fast foods.

While many sources of sugar are obvious, such as candy, cake, and sodas, there are hidden sources in processed foods and non-food products.

Sugar is used not only to sweeten foods. It is also used as a preservative, thickener, and a baking aid. Sugar is used to retain the color in ketchup. It is added to baked goods for yeast growth and to give a golden color to the crusts. In soft drinks, it adds mass. In chewing gum, it adds texture and pliability. Raw potatoes in restaurants are dipped in sugar water before frying to give them crispness. Refined sugar is added to tobacco to enhance the flavor and burning quality.

Aside from table sugar (sucrose), food manufacturers call sugar by many other names. Knowledge of these names on product labels can help you to shop and compare the sugar content of various food products. Avoid or limit foods that list any of these other names for sugar among the first three ingredients on the food label, which indicates that the product contains a large amount.

The following is a list of some of the sugars that may be added to foods.

- **Brown sugar** is sucrose (white sugar) colored with molasses syrup.
- **Confectioner's sugar** is powdered sugar with cornstarch added to prevent lumping and crystallization.
- **Dextrose**, known as glucose or corn sugar, is made from cornstarch.
- **Demerara** sugar is a raw sugar that has been purified, and is often described as natural, unrefined cane sugar.
- **Fructose** or levulose "fruit sugar" is a naturally occurring sugar found in honey and in fruits and other parts of plants.
- **Fruit juice concentrates**; fruits are concentrated through heat and enzyme treatments and filtration, which remove fiber, flavor, and nutrients. A fruit juice sweetener is identical in calories, sugar, and nutrients to sugar syrups.
- **High fructose corn syrup (HFCS)** is made from the breakdown of cornstarch, which results in a mixture of dextrose and fructose.

- **Honey** is a mixture of sugar formed from nectar by the enzyme invetose, which is present in the body of a bee. Honey varies in composition depending on the source of the nectar (clover, orange blossom, sage, etc.). Raw unprocessed honey, unlike sugar, provides small amounts of minerals. It has more carbohydrates and calories than granulated sugar, and it is sweeter.

  One teaspoon of honey = 17 carbs and 64 calories.
  One teaspoon of sugar = 13 carbs and 50 calories.

- **Invert sugar** is a liquid sweetener that results from converting sucrose to a mixture of glucose and fructose.

- **Molasses** is syrup left from processing cane or beet sugar. Darker molasses and blackstrap molasses is superior in providing small amounts of vitamins and minerals.

- **Raw sugar** is what's left after processing sugarcane to remove molasses and refined white sugar. It is actually not "raw" and has been processed and refined. According to the U.S. Food and Drug Administration, raw sugar is "unfit for direct use as food or as a food ingredient because it requires additional purification."

- **Sucrose** is white, refined table sugar made from sugarcane or sugar beets.

- **Turbinado** is raw sugar that has been steam cleaned to a light tan color.

All sugars should be used in moderation by most healthy people, and sparingly by people with low calorie needs such as those with diabetes.

Sugar substitutes

Sugar substitutes, also called artificial or non-nutritive sweeteners, are another option for sweetening your food. They can be helpful when used in a weight management program, diabetes meal planning, and reducing the risk of tooth decay. However, if you use sugar substitutes you should be aware that there has been controversy regarding potential health threats.

The following is a list of a few common sugar substitutes and sweeteners.

- **Acesulfame potassium (Acesulfame-K)** is 200 times sweeter than sugar. It is found under the names of Sunnett, Sweet & Safe, Sweet One, and Ace-K. It contains no calories and heating does not reduce its sweetening power.
- **Aspartame** is 200 times sweeter than sugar. It is found under the names of NutraSweet and Equal. Each gram of aspartame contains 4 calories, however, the amount needed to sweeten foods is very tiny, so the amount of calories is of no consequence. There have been controversial studies indicating that this sweetener can cause brain neurological disorders, but the FDA has concluded that the data from these studies were inconclusive. However, many consumers, as well as scientists, are not convinced that long-term daily intake of aspartame is completely safe. Aspartame is known to be dangerous for people with phenylketonuria (PKU), a genetic disorder in which the body lacks the enzyme necessary to metabolize phenylalanine (an essential amino acid), one of the two compounds used to make aspartame. In addition, aspartame is not recom-

mended for use by pregnant or women who are breastfeeding.

• **Polyols or sugar alcohols** are found under the names of mannitol, xlitol, erythitol, D-tagatose, isomalt, lactitol, maltitol, trahalose, polyglycitol, polyglucitol, and sorbital. Sugar alcohols don't actually contain sugar or alcohol, but they are a type of carbohydrate, and they produce some glucose in the blood. Because sugar alcohols are not technically a form of sugar, manufacturers can advertise their food products as "sugar-free." However, this does not mean that the product is "carbohydrate free" or "low calorie." They contain 0.2 to 3 calories per gram. If you have diabetes, you must keep in mind that sugar alcohol counts as carbohydrates, even though the amount of calories is less than table sugar. And if you are trying to lose weight, unless you reduce the total calories you eat, the use of sugar substitutes will not help you to lose weight.

• **Saccharin** is 200 to 700 times sweeter than sugar and is found under the names of Sweet 'N Low, Sugar Twin, Sweet 'N Low Brown, Necta Sweet, and Hermeasatas. It contains 0 calories per gram. Numerous scientific studies over the years have found that saccharin causes malignant tumors (cancer) in animals. There has been a great deal of controversy over the use of saccharin, and in the 1970's the FDA proposed a ban on its use in the United States. But, after much controversy, years of review, and public pressure, the FDA formally withdrew its proposal to ban saccharin's use. Since 1977, however, all foods containing saccharin must carry the following label: *"Use of this product may be hazardous to your health. This prod-*

uct contains saccharin, which has been determined to cause cancer in laboratory animals."

- **Splenda** (Sucralose) is 600 times sweeter than sugar. It is the only artificial sweetener that is made from sugar. It contains 0 calories per gram. The body does not recognize sucralose as a sugar or a carbohydrate so it does not metabolize it, making it suitable for those with diabetes.
- **Stevia** (Stevioside) is 250 to 300 times sweeter than sugar, and is also called sweetleaf. Stevia is a non-caloric herb that is native to subtropical and tropical South America and Central America. While stevia has been used as a sweetener for centuries in other countries, the FDA has not approved it as a sweetener in the United States. This is why it is not on the supermarket shelves with NutraSweet and other sweeteners. However, it is sold in the U.S. as a dietary supplement and can be found in health food stores.

Healthy options for reducing sugar in your diet

- Buy unsweetened cereals or sweeten cereals by adding fresh fruits such as banana slices or a few raisins.
- Avoid granola bars and most sports bars.
- Drink fresh fruit juices, herb teas, and water.
- Avoid sweetened fruit juices, soda, and punch.
- Eat fruit that is not canned in heavy syrups.
- Avoid prepackaged mixes, which are high in sugar.
- Reduce the amount of sugar called for in your favorite recipes.
- Try different spices such as cinnamon, coriander, and ginger to bring out the natural sweet flavor of

foods.

- Eat fruits for desserts more often, instead of cakes, cookies, pies or candy. Fruits satisfy sweet cravings and provide healthful nutrition and fiber along with the sweet taste.
- Limit dried fruits.
- Eat your fruits whole as much as possible instead of juicing them, unless you are fasting. A juicer removes the pulp which contains the fiber and vitamins, leaving mostly concentrated sugars and calories.

  If you use a blender to make juice, the pulp or fiber are retained in the juice. However, blenders operate at high speed, producing only a small amount of liquid. In order to drink the juice, water must be added.

- Refined sugars should not make up more than 10 percent of your diet.

CHAPTER 18

Don't Shake the Salt

African Americans eat entirely too much salt! And unfortunately many of us continue to do so until otherwise advised by a physician. At this point serious consequences are already underway.

The worst consequence of heavy salt (sodium) consumption is that it raises your blood pressure. High blood pressure (hypertension) is no stranger to the African American community. One out of three African Americans suffers from high blood pressure. I shouldn't need to remind you of the dangers of hypertension, but I must. It is the leading cause of heart attacks, strokes, kidney disease, and eye problems (blindness) in the black community, and is responsible for 20 percent of the African American deaths in the United States.

Hypertension is defined as systolic blood pressure of 140 or higher (the upper number in a blood pressure reading), or a diastolic blood pressure of 90 or higher (the bottom number in a blood pressure reading). Pre-hypertension is when the systolic blood pressure is 120 to 139, and the diastolic is 80 to 89.

During one of my jobs as a registered nurse, I was responsible for checking blood pressure in a predomi-nately African American community. I would go to vari-ous community centers, senior citizen centers, or some-times set up my blood pressure station in front of a bank.

I found people with blood pressures as high as 220/120, and had to refer them to a doctor. Some were subsequently hospitalized. Keep in mind that these were individuals walking around tending to their usual daily activities, not knowing they were in danger of having a stroke.

Many people still believe in the myth that you can feel when your blood pressure is rising. However, this is not the case. Sometimes people with high blood pressure do not have any symptoms. This is what makes hyperten-sion so dangerous and why it is called the "silent killer."

Another common myth is that you cannot get high blood pressure if you are not overweight. I encountered many people who had high blood pressure and were not overweight. For example, one of the ladies that I referred to the hospital because her blood pressure was danger-ously high, was very slim and had never had a weight problem.

Cutting back on the amount of salt that you eat will help to control your blood pressure, and lower the amount of fluid (water) you hold in your body—a condi-tion called "edema." Extra fluid in your body causes a strain on your heart and kidneys and raises your blood pressure.

Where are we getting all this salt?

Seventy-seven percent of the salt in your diet comes from what we eat in restaurants, or from processed foods such as canned soups, luncheon meats, cured meats, frozen foods, potato chips and commercial baked products. The rest comes from the salt added at the table, and salt added while cooking.

Salt is used by manufactures to preserve food, and also to improve the taste and texture of food. Salted foods such as soups seem thicker and less watery. Salt increases sweetness in products such as soft drinks, cookies and cakes. Salt helps cover up any metallic or chemical aftertaste in products such as soft drinks. Salt even decreases dryness in foods such as crackers and pretzels.

Even if you limit the salt added to your food, the food itself may already be high in sodium.

It is recommended that you consume less than 2,300 mg (approximately 1 teaspoon) of salt per day. Individuals with high blood pressure, particularly African Americans, middle-aged and older adults, should consume no more than 1,500 mg per day (¾ of a teaspoon).

Unfortunately, the average American consumes 4,000 mg to 6,000 mg of sodium per day (2 to 3 teaspoons). This is two or three times the amount that is recommended. Given the amount of sodium that is already added to prepared food, consuming excessive amounts can occur too easily.

The following are example of foods high in sodium:

Bacon Bits	Mustards
Barbeque sauce	Olives
Bouillon cubes	Onion salt
Catsup	Pickles
Celery salt	Salad dressing
Cocktail sauce	Salsa
Gravy (canned or mix)	Soy, tamari sauce
Marinades	Steak sauce
Meat tenderizer	Worcestershire sauce

Additionally, the following are hidden sources of sodium that are not counted in the sodium content of food:

- Baking power and baking soda - leavening agents
- Monosodium glutamate (MSG) - flavor enhancer
- Sodium alginate - makes chocolate milk and ice cream smooth
- Sodium benzoate - preservative
- Sodium citrate - buffer, controls acidity in soft drinks and fruit drinks
- Sodium nitrate - curing agent in meat & sausages, provides color, and prevents botulism disease
- Sodium sulfite - bleach fruits for artificial coloring and preservative in prunes

Ways to reduce sodium in your diet

- Eat fewer processed foods and snacks such as potato chips and frozen foods.
- Eat less cured meats, ham, bacon, hot dogs, sausages, and processed luncheon meats.

- Eat plain fresh or frozen vegetables instead of canned.
- Prepare low sodium meals.
- Rinse canned foods, such as tuna, to remove some sodium.
- Don't add salt when cooking rice, pasta, or other foods.
- Choose foods labeled low, reduced, or sodium free.
- Use herbs and spices, lemon juice, lime juice, and vinegar to flavor foods instead of salt.
- Taste your food before adding salt.
- Decrease the amount of salt in recipes.
- Read food labels for sodium content.

Instead of adding salt, exercise your option to enhance your food with healthy herbs and spices, learning new and exciting ways to reduce your sodium intake.

ENHANCING FOOD FLAVOR WITH HERBS AND SPICES

HERB OR SPICE	FLAVOR	USE TO ENHANCE
ALLSPICE	Combination of clove, cinnamon, and nutmeg	Chicken, fish, meat, pasta curries, desserts
BASIL	Mild peppery flavor with a trace of mint and clove	Tomato sauces, pasta, chicken, fish, Italian dishes, salad
CARAWAY SEEDS	Nutty, licorice flavor	Cooked vegetables such as cabbage, broccoli, carrots, potatoes, squash
CHIVES	Mild, sweet onion taste	Salad, omelets, potatoes, pasta, seafood, meats
CINNAMON	Sweet, woody flavor	Sweet potatoes, squash, apples, desserts
CUMIN	Nutty flavor and aroma	Curried vegetables, fish, poultry, and beans
CURRY	A blend of spices: cumin, pepper, chili peppers, ginger, onion, cinnamon, paprika, cilantro, turmeric	Lamb, meat-based dishes, soups, eggs, fish
DILL (FRESH)	Slightly sweet with sharp tangy flavor	Fish, chicken, carrots, beets, cauliflower, spinach, green beans, tomatoes, potatoes

HERB OR SPICE	FLAVOR	USE TO ENHANCE
GARLIC	Strong, pungent	Meat, fish, poultry, salads, sauces, soups
GINGER	Sweet flavor with a hint of citrus	Rice, chicken, and marinades
MARJORAM	Mild oregano taste, with a minty, basil flavor	Eggplant, tomato-based dishes, fish, meat, poultry, eggs, vegetables
OREGANO	Pungent, somewhat sweet and peppery flavor	Italian cuisine, tomatoes, mushrooms, poultry, lentils
PARSLEY	Green gentle flavor	Chicken, fish, pasta, potatoes, garnish
ROSEMARY	Piney flavor	Meat, fish, poultry, sauces, stews, vegetables, stuffing
SAGE	Musty flavor	Bread, stuffing, potatoes, chicken, duck, pork, eggplant, beans stews, soups
TARRAGON	Mild licorice flavor	Chicken, fish, vegetables, eggs, salad dressings, tomatoes, mushrooms, carrots
THYME	Somewhat bitter with a minty-clove like flavor	Poultry, salad dressing, dried beans, soups, eggplant, mushrooms, potatoes, summer squash
TURMERIC	Sharp, woodsy taste	Indian cuisine, potatoes, light-colored vegetables

CHAPTER 19

Supplement Wisely

To supplement or not to supplement; it's a question that many people wonder about. The answer is simple. Supplements such as multivitamins/minerals should be used to enhance your diet, not to replace it. A standard multivitamin supplement can only compliment your diet—it doesn't come close to making up for an unhealthy diet. Hence the word "supplement."

An orange, for example, provides beta-carotene, calcium, folate, and other nutrients, while a vitamin C supplement basically provides vitamin C, and does not contain these important nutrients. (See food sources of vitamins and minerals at the end of this section.)

Having said that, there are a number of good reasons why multivitamins and minerals are beneficial and should be used to compliment your diet:

- You may be eating too many processed foods that are depleted of nutrients, further destroying the value of foods through overcooking and harmful additives.
- You may not be eating enough, or including a variety of well-balanced foods in your diet.
- Your doctor may have recommended a specific vitamin supplement for a health problem.

Let me caution you that taking mega doses of certain vitamins and minerals can be harmful. Fat-soluble vitamins A, D, E, and K unused by your body after digestion are stored in the fat of your body, and liver. Therefore, an excess amount of these vitamins can accumulate in your blood stream and become toxic without you realizing it. For example, you may be taking several supplements that contain Vitamin A: a vitamin A tablet to help improve your eyesight, a daily multivitamin tablet to supplement your diet, and an herbal supplement tablet for a cold. Heavy doses of vitamin A can cause headaches, hair loss, dry skin, joint pain, and vomiting.

Conversely, water-soluble vitamin C, and the seven B vitamins (B-1, B-2, B-3, B-5, B-6, B-9, and B-12) dissolve in water and are not stored in your body in any significant amounts. If you take too much, water-soluble vitamins are typically excreted in your urine. However, there are exceptions. For example, taking large doses of vitamin B-6 (over 150 milligrams/day which is taken commonly for premenstrual syndrome) has been associated with neurological symptoms (twitching, numbness, etc.), chest pain, and muscle weakness.

The toxic effects of some minerals are a concern as well. For example large doses of zinc can produce chills, fever, heartburn, indigestion, nausea, sore throat, and unusual tiredness.

I suggest that you consult with your doctor or nutritionist regarding your individual supplement needs.

VITAMIN FOOD SOURCES

VITAMINS	HEALTH BENEFITS	NATURAL FOOD SOURCES
VITAMIN A	Essential for night vision, healthy skin, hair, mucous membranes, and resistance to infection	Apricots, bok choy, dried peaches, asparagus, beets, greens, broccoli, cantaloupe, carrots, collards, garlic, kale, papayas, peaches, pumpkins, red peppers, spirulina, spinach, sweet potatoes, Swiss chard, turnip greens, watercress, yellow squash, milk, fish liver oils, whole egg, liver, milk products
VITAMIN B1 (THIAMIN)	Essential for metabolism of carbohydrates; muscle tone, nerve function, digestion, appetite, elimination	Legumes, potatoes, breads, cereals, brown rice, fish, meats, egg yolks, poultry, rice, bran, wheat germ, whole grains, asparagus, brewer's yeast, oatmeal, nuts, plums, dried prunes, raisins, peanuts, spirulina, watercress
VITAMIN B2 (RIBOFLAVIN)	Convert fats, carbohydrates and proteins into energy; healthy eyes, skin, and mucous membranes	Green leafy vegetables, breads, cereals, eggs, milk and milk products, egg yolk, fish, meat, poultry, whole grains, asparagus, avocados, broccoli, Brussels sprouts, currants, dandelion greens, dulse, kelp, mushrooms, molasses, nuts, watercress

VITAMINS	HEALTH BENEFITS	NATURAL FOOD SOURCES
VITAMIN B3 (NIACIN)	Essential for protein, fat, carbohydrate metabolism; nervous system function; appetite, digestion	Broccoli, carrots, dandelion greens, cheese, corn flour, dates, eggs, fish, milk, peanuts, meat, brewer's yeast, potatoes, tomatoes, wheat germ, whole wheat products, breads, peas, beans
VITAMIN B6 (PYRIDOXINE)	Essential for helping to convert protein into energy	Brewer's yeast, carrots, chicken, eggs, fish, meat, peas, spinach, sunflower seeds, walnuts, wheat germ
VITAMIN B9 (FOLIC ACID)	Essential for formation of red blood cells, functioning of intestines, protein metabolism	Dark green leafy vegetables, asparagus, turnips, beets, Brussels sprouts, lima beans, soybeans, mung beans, white beans, beef liver, meats, fish, brewer's yeast, whole grains, orange juice, avocados, milk
VITAMIN B12	Essential for red blood cell formation, growth, and a healthy nervous system	Green leafy vegetables, meat, fish, eggs
VITAMIN C (ASCORBIC ACID)	Essential for healthy bones, teeth, skin, and gums; wound healing; energy production; resistance to infection	Citrus fruits, tomatoes, green vegetables, asparagus, avocados, beet greens, black currants, broccoli, Brussels sprouts, cantaloupe, collards, dandelion greens, dulse, kale, mangos, mustard greens, onions, oranges, papayas, green peas, sweet peppers, persimmons, pineapple, radishes, rose hips, strawberries, melons

VITAMINS	HEALTH BENEFITS	NATURAL FOOD SOURCES
VITAMIN D	Essential for healthy bones, teeth, and for calcium absorption	Fish liver oils, fatty saltwater fish, dairy products, butter, oatmeal, sweet potatoes, vegetable oils; exposure to sunlight
VITAMIN E	Essential for normal reproduction; formation of red blood cells; muscle function	Green leafy vegetables, vegetable oils, legumes, nuts, seeds, whole grains, brown rice, organ meats, soybeans, sweet potatoes, watercress, wheat, wheat germ
VITAMIN K	Essential for blood clotting	Dark green leafy vegetables, soybean, vegetable oils, eggs, margarine, liver, asparagus, blackstrap molasses, broccoli, Brussels sprouts, cabbage, cauliflower, egg yolk, liver, oatmeal, rye, safflower oil, wheat

MINERAL FOOD SOURCES

MINERAL	HEALTH BENEFITS	NATURAL FOOD SOURCES
POTASSIUM	Essential for regulating fluids inside cells-along with sodium; nerve impulse transmission; muscle contractions; maintenance of normal blood pressure	Fresh fruits, dried fruits, vegetables, meats, legumes, nuts, seeds
MAGNESIUM	Essential for maintaining acid-alkaline balance and healthy functioning of nerves and muscles; activates enzymes to metabolize blood sugars, proteins, and carbohydrates	Seeds, unrefined grains, beans, green vegetables, nuts, figs, seafood, molasses, yellow corn, coconut, apples
PHOSPHORUS	Essential for the formation of bones and teeth; use of proteins, fats, and carbohydrates; nerve and muscle function	Nuts, poultry, milk and milk products, eggs, fish, grains, nuts, legumes
SODIUM	Essential for fluid balance; nerve and muscle function	Almost all foods in varying amounts
IRON	Essential for transporting oxygenated blood through the body; synthesis of collagen, functioning of the immune system.	Green leafy vegetables, meat, fish, beans, molasses, kelp, brewer's yeast, broccoli, and seeds
IODINE	Essential for development and functioning of the thyroid gland; growth; metabolism	Seafood, vegetables, iodized salt
CHROMIUM	Essential for glucose tolerance; works with insulin for controlling blood sugar	Brewer's yeast, beef, liver, eggs, chicken, oysters, green peppers, wheat germ, apples, bananas and spinach

MINERAL	HEALTH BENEFITS	NATURAL FOOD SOURCES
COPPER	Essential for absorption and utilization of zinc and iron	Whole grains, nuts, shell-fish, liver, dark-green leafy vegetables
SELENIUM	Functions closely with vitamin E and supports critical antioxidant enzyme functions	Seafood, organ meats, grains, vegetables
ZINC	Essential for muscle formation; functioning of enzymes; supports the immune system; normal synthesis of protein; and health of the reproductive organs.	Beans, whole grains, pumpkin seeds, meat, fish, mushrooms

CHAPTER 20

Turn on the Water Works

Drinking enough water on a daily basis is one of the most important things we can do to improve and maintain health. Human beings need water in order to survive and thrive. Without water a person can't survive more than eight to ten days.

Did you know your body is made up of 65 to 70 percent water? If you don't drink enough water your organs will suffer drastically.

There are numerous benefits to drinking water. Water circulates through your blood and lymphatic system, transporting oxygen and nutrients to cells, and removing wastes through urine, feces, and sweat. It softens your skin, increases your energy, provides lubrication and cushioning to your joints, and softens tissues. Without water, you could not digest or absorb the foods you eat or eliminate your body's digestive waste.

Lack of water can lead to dehydration, a condition that occurs when you don't have enough water in your body to carry on normal functions. It only takes a loss of 1 or 2 percent of your body's total water content to cause dehydration.

Actually, when you feel thirsty, you are already suffering from slight dehydration, so you should not wait until you are thirsty to drink water. Even mild dehydration can sap your energy and make you tired. Severe dehydration is a serious medical condition that requires immediate attention.

Some of the signs of dehydration:

- Excessive thirst
- Fatigue
- Headache
- Dry mouth
- Little or no urination
- Muscle weakness
- Dizziness
- Lightheadedness

It takes an average of 8 to 10 glasses of water to replenish the fluids our bodies lose each day. How much water a person needs depends largely on the volume of urine, feces, and sweat excreted daily.

If you engage in an activity that makes you sweat, such as physical exercise, you'll need to drink extra water to make up for the fluid that you lost. If you are ill, and experiencing diarrhea or vomiting, you will need extra water to replenish what was lost. In hot and humid weather, extra water is needed to lower your body temperature and protect against dehydration.

For your body to function normally, you need to replace the water you lose by consuming beverages and foods that contain water. For example, fruits and vegetables are 80-90 percent water, meats are made up of 50 percent water, and grains, such as oats and rice, can have as much as 35 percent water. However, drinking plain water remains the most effective and least expensive way to replace lost fluids from your body.

It is best to drink non-caffeinated and non-alcoholic beverages because caffeine and alcohol increase your output of urine, which can result in dehydrating your body. Some people prefer soft drinks, fruit juice, and sports drinks. Although these liquids may quench your thirst for fluids, they typically are high in sugar and calories and do little to reduce thirst.

Types of Water

Tap water, also referred to as municipal water or public drinking water, is drawn directly from a faucet or spigot. The U.S. Environmental Protection Agency (EPA) regulates tap water in terms of production, distribution, and quality.

Bottled water, which has become hugely popular, is regulated by the U.S. Food and Drug Administration (FDA). The FDA monitors and inspects bottled water products and processing plants under its general food safety program.

Bottled water may be used as an ingredient in beverages, such as diluted juices or flavored water drinks.

However, beverages labeled as containing "sparkling water," "seltzer water," "soda water," "tonic water," or "club soda" are not included as bottled water under the FDA regulations. These beverages may contain sugar and calories and are classified as soft drinks.

Is bottled water better for you than tap water? Well, the experts are still debating this question. However, since both are being regulated and monitored for safety and quality, it's up to you to make your own decision, possibly based on cost versus taste.

Many people prefer bottled water for its taste. Chlorine is often used to disinfect tap water and can leave an aftertaste. Some bottled water manufacturers use ozonation, a form of supercharged oxygen, and/or ultraviolet light, as the final disinfecting agent, neither of which leaves an aftertaste.

Types of bottled water

- **Spring water**: This is bottled water collected from springs; it can only be obtained from the spring itself or an underground source feeding into the spring.
- **Mineral water:** It is generally obtained from a natural spring or underground source, and the manufacturer does not modify the mineral content. The dissolved solids that it contains give it a distinctive taste and body.
- **Purified water:** Tap water that has been treated before bottling by distillation or reverse osmosis, both of which are processes that remove minerals from the water. The resulting water is the highest purity but the taste is often considered 'bland' or 'flat'.

- **Sparkling water:** Water that has had carbon dioxide added to it. The carbon dioxide bubbles out of the water when you expose it to air. Sparkling waters may be labeled as "sparkling drinking water," "sparkling mineral water," "sparkling spring water," etc.

Healthy options for drinking water

- Upon rising, before breakfast, drink two glasses of water at room temperature with freshly squeezed lemon in it. It will help you feel better and more energized. And, it will help you to shed some of yesterday's leftover waste.
- Don't drink water or liquids with your meals. Drink 30 minutes before a meal and wait 45 minutes to an hour after meals. This will avoid diluting your important digestive enzymes.
- Keep water within reach, at home, in your car, or at work, to keep you hydrated throughout the day. It will also help you avoid unhealthy beverages that falsely cure thirst.
- Take water breaks. Mid-afternoon is a good time to take a break and have a bottle of water.
- Drink a glass of water after having beverages with caffeine or alcohol, to keep from being dehydrated.
- Increase your intake of fresh fruits and vegetables, which have a high water content as well as other health benefits.

Lottie Mallory-Perkins

*"People respond to information
in their own time,
and according to their own needs.
Once you plant the seed,
your job is done.
The seed must be allowed to cultivate
at its own rate."*

Author's Note

If you have reached this page in the book, I would like to say… *congratulations*! You have taken a quantum leap toward improving your overall health and the health of the African American community.

But please, do not stop here. Your next step is to incorporate all that you have learned into your daily routine.

As you make your healthy lifestyle choices, I will remain with you in spirit.

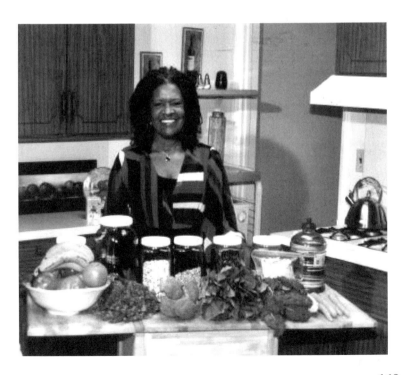

References and Resources

Bad Blood: The Tuskegee Syphilis Experiment, a Tragedy of Race and Medicine, by James H. Jones, The Free Press, New York, 1981.

Bad Meat and Brown Bananas: Building a Legacy of Health by Confronting Health Disparities Around Food, by David C. Sloane, for the African American Building a Legacy of Health Coalition/REACH 2010 Project, Journal of General Internal Medicine, July 2003.

Black Americans Less Likely to Recognize Overweight and Obesity, Gary Bennett PhD and Kathleen Y. Wolin ScD, Dana-Farber Cancer Institute, News Release, December 2006.

Black or African American Population, The Centers of Disease Control and Prevention, Office of Communication, July 1, 2005.

Body Mass Index BMI, National Institute of Health, www.nhlbi.nih. gov/guidelines/obesity/bmi_tbi.htm

The Black Women's Health Book: Speaking for Ourselves, Edited by Evelyn C. White, Seal Press, Seattle, Washington, 1994.

Closing the Gap: Reducing Health Disparities Affecting African Americans, U.S. Department of Health and Human Services, November 19, 2001.

Childhood Obesity in the United States: Facts and Figures, Institute of Medicine, September 2004.

Comparison of the Atkins, Ornish, LEARN, and Zone Diets for Change in weight and related risk factors among overweight premenopausal women, The Journal of American Medical Association Vol. 297. No. 9, March 7, 2007.

A Consumers Dictionary of Food Additives, by Ruth Winter, The Three Rivers Press, New York, 1999.

Dietary Guidelines for Americans: Department of Health and Human Services and Department of Agriculture, January 12, 2005.

Eat 5 to 9 a Day for Better Health Program: The National Cancer Institute.

Eliminating Racial and Ethnic Disparities, The Centers of Disease Control and Prevention, Office of Minority Health, July 1, 2005.

Health of Black or African American Population, The National Center for Health Statistics, 2000-2002.

How To Be Your Own Nutritionist, by Stuart Berger, Avon Books, New York, 1998.

Health and Healing, by Andrew Weil, Houghton Mifflin Company, Boston, 1995.

Health Disparities Experience by Black or African Americans — United States, The Centers of Disease Control and Prevention, MMWR, January 14, 2005/54(01):1-3.

Health Insurance Coverage and Access to Care Among African Americans, Kaiser Commission on Medicaid and the Uninsured, June, 2000.

How to Understand and Use Nutritional Facts Labels, U.S. Food and Drug Administration, November, 2004.

Learned Optimism: How to Change Your Mind and Your Life, by Martin E. Seligman, Free Press, New York, 1998.

More Supermarkets Linked to Healthier Diets, American Journal of Public Health, by Dr. Steven B. Wing and Anna Diez Roux, November 2002.

Nutrition and Overweight, U.S. Department of Health and Human Services. Public Health Services, Healthy People 2010, Progress Review, January 21, 2004.

Risk Factors and Interventions for Obesity in African-American Women, Journal of Multicultural Nursing & Health, by Sharon Aneta Bryant and Martha Neff Smith, Winter 2001.

Stress Management, by Wendy Ruthstiver, Homestead Schools, Inc. 1999.

United States Life Tables, 2003, Volume 54, Number 14, April 19, 2006, National Center for Health Statistics, Centers for Disease Control.

What to Say When You Talk to Yourself, by Shad Helmsteller, Pocket Books, New York, 1982.

American Heart Association
800-242-8721
www.americanheart.org

American Diabetes Association
800-342-2383
www.diabetes.org/community

The American Cancer Society
800-ACS-2345
www.cancer.org

Black Women Health
www.blackwomenhealth.com

African American Health Care & Medical Information
www.BlackHealthCare.com

Centers for Disease Control and Prevention
800-311-3435
www.cdc.gov

Health Finders
Healthfinders@nhic.org
P.O. Box 1133, Washington, DC 200013-113

Medline Plus
www.medlineplus.com

The McKinley Health Center at the University of Illinois
mckinley.uiuc.edu/multiculturalhealth/aboutus.html

The National Cancer Institute
www.cancer.gov

The National Library of Medicine
301-496-4000
www.nlm.nih.gov/medlineplus/africanamericanhealth.html

The National Institute of Diabetes and Digestive and Kidney Diseases
202-828-1025
win@info.niddk.nih.gov

The National Heart, Lung, and Blood Institute
301-592-8573
www.nhlbi.nih.gov

The U.S. Food and Drug Administration
FDA's food label information on the web:
www.cfsan.fda.gov
FDA's Food Safety Hotline: 800-332-4010

About the Author

Lottie Perkins has been in the health care industry for the past 37 years. She holds a Bachelor's Degree in Nursing from UCLA, and a Master's Degree in Health Administration from the University of La Verne, and is a Certified Natural Health Consultant through the Clayton School of Holistic Health. She is a successful entrepreneur, and president of her own business, *Perkins Enterprises: Health Consultation and Training.*

Through work experience and her private practice, she has had the opportunity to lecture and conduct workshops on preventative health, healthy lifestyle choices, and stress management. In addition, she has an extensive background as an instructor in nurse assistant training programs, and as a consultant to health care agencies.

Her true passion is helping people to make healthy lifestyle choices. By this she means doing whatever it takes to be healthy. She has lived a holistic lifestyle of meditation, prayer, exercise, and vegetarian eating for many years. This has proven to be a great benefit in her life and to her overall health.

In this book, she shares her knowledge, insight, and personal experiences to help other African Americans recognize the benefits of making conscious lifestyle choices that increase their quality of life.